Elizabeth Podnieks, EdD, RN
Jordan I. Kosberg, PhD, ACSW
Ariela Lowenstein, PhD
Editors

Elder Abuse: Selected Papers from the Prague World Congress on Family Violence

Elder Abuse: Selected Papers from the Prague World Congress on Family Violence has been co-published simultaneously as *Journal of Elder Abuse & Neglect*, Volume 15, Numbers 3/4 2003.

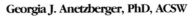

Pre-publication REVIEWS, COMMENTARIES, EVALUATIONS . . .

"The editors are to be commended. . . . SOME OF THE CONTENT IS GROUNDBREAKING, covering topics little investigated in the past, such as the abuse of grandparents or elder abuse awareness and response in faith communities."

Georgia J. Anetzberger, PhD, ACSW
Assistant Professor
of Health Care Administration
Cleveland State University

HMTP

The Haworth Maltreatment & Trauma Press®
An Imprint of The Haworth Press, Inc.

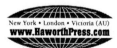

New York • London • Victoria (AU)
www.HaworthPress.com

Elder Abuse:
Selected Papers
from the Prague
World Congress
on Family Violence

Elder Abuse: Selected Papers from the Prague World Congress on Family Violence has been co-published simultaneously as *Journal of Elder Abuse & Neglect*, Volume 15, Numbers 3/4 2003.

The *Journal of Elder Abuse & Neglect*™ Monographic "Separates"

Below is a list of "separates," which in serials librarianship means a special issue simultaneously published as a special journal issue or double-issue *and* as a "separate" hardbound monograph. (This is a format which we also call a "DocuSerial.")

"Separates" are published because specialised libraries or professionals may wish to purchase a specific thematic issue by itself in a format which can be separately cataloged and shelved, as opposed to purchasing the journal on an on-going basis. Faculty members may also more easily consider a "separate" for classroom adoption.

"Separates" are carefully classified separately with the major book jobbers so that the journal tie-in can be noted on new book order slips to avoid duplicate purchasing.

You may wish to visit Haworth's website at . . .

http://www.HaworthPress.com

. . . to search our online catalog for complete tables of contents of these separates and related publications.

You may also call 1-800-HAWORTH (outside US/Canada: 607-722-5857), or Fax 1-800-895-0582 (outside US/Canada: 607-771-0012), or e-mail at:

docdelivery@haworthpress.com

Elder Abuse: Selected Papers from the Prague World Congress on Family Violence, edited by Elizabeth Podnieks, EdD, RN, Jordan I. Kosberg, PhD, ACSW, and Ariela Lowenstein, PhD, (Vol. 15, No. 3/4, 2003). *Elder Abuse: Selected Papers from the Prague World Congress on Family Violence is an invaluable collection of the most important presentation papers from the Prague World Congress on Family Violence. International experts use a multidisciplinary approach to present the latest research and detailed information on the difficult issues involving elder abuse in various countries around the world, as well as useful ideas and revealing insights to help provide practical strategies for dealing with the numerous facets of this disturbing issue. This comprehensive source is richly referenced with helpful tables to clearly explain data.*

Self-Neglect, edited by James G. O'Brien, MD (Vol. 11, No. 2, 1999). *Through case studies, this informative book explores the ways in which patients practice self-neglect by not taking medicine, extreme lack of self-care, refusal to eat, failure to comply with a medical regimen, and alcohol abuse and offers ways to identify and understand this dangerous behavior and offer your patients better care for this condition.*

Elder Abuse and Neglect in Residential Settings: Different National Backgrounds and Similar Responses, edited by Frank Glendenning, PhD, and Paul Kingston, PhD (Vol. 10, No. 1/2, 1999). *Gain insights from countries where elder abuse and neglect have been recognized as an issue requiring social policy attention.*

Elder Mistreatment: Ethical Issues, Dilemmas, and Decisions, edited by Tanya Fusco Johnson, PhD, MDiv (Vol. 7, No. 2/3, 1995). *"I recommend this book to members of all health fields. It covers in depth the major ethical topics of autonomy, beneficence, legal competence, and justice, yet remains practical by discussing constraints to ideal solutions. Physical therapists who practice in-home care and in nursing homes would find special benefit." (Physical Therapy)*

Elder Abuse: International and Cross-Cultural Perspectives, edited by Jordan I. Kosberg, PhD, and Juanita L. Garcia, EdD (Vol. 6, No. 3/4, 1995). *"A welcome and original contribution to the literature on elder abuse and is recommended reading for all with an interest in this field." (Age & Aging)*

Protecting Judgement-Impaired Adults: Issues, Interventions, and Policies, edited by Edmund F. Dejowski, JD, PhD (Vol. 2, No. 3/4, 1990). *"Provides eye-opening information about guardianship and alternative methods of serving judgement-impaired adults. . . . practical guidelines and suggestions for professional and nonprofessionals who find themselves involved with this population." (Adultspan)*

Elder Abuse: Selected Papers from the Prague World Congress on Family Violence

Elizabeth Podnieks, EdD, RN
Jordan I. Kosberg PhD, ACSW
Ariela Lowenstein, PhD
Editors

Elder Abuse: Selected Papers from the Prague World Congress on Family Violence has been co-published simultaneously as *Journal of Elder Abuse & Neglect*, Volume 15, Numbers 3/4 2003.

HMTP

The Haworth Maltreatment & Trauma Press®
An Imprint of The Haworth Press, Inc.

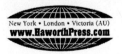

New York • London • Victoria (AU)
www.HaworthPress.com

Published by

The Haworth Maltreatment & Trauma Press, 10 Alice Street, Binghamton, NY 13904-1580 USA

The Haworth Maltreatment & Trauma Press is an imprint of The Haworth Press, Inc., 10 Alice Street, Binghamton, NY 13904-1580 USA.

Elder Abuse: Selected Papers from the Prague World Congress on Family Violence has been co-published simultaneously as *Journal of Elder Abuse & Neglect*, Volume 15, Numbers 3/4 2003.

The development, preparation, and publication of this work has been undertaken with great care. However, the publisher, employees, editors, and agents of The Haworth Press and all imprints of The Haworth Press, Inc., including The Haworth Medical Press® and Pharmaceutical Products Press®, are not responsible for any errors contained herein or for consequences that may ensue from use of materials or information contained in this work. Opinions expressed by the author(s) are not necessarily those of The Haworth Press, Inc.

Cover design by Kerry E. Mack.

Library of Congress Cataloging-in-Publication Data

Prague World Congress on Family Violence (2003: Prague, Czech Republic)
  Elder abuse: selected papers from the Prague World congress on Family Violence/Elizabeth Podnieks, Jordan I. Kosberg, Ariela Lowenstein, editors.
      p. cm.
  Papers presented at the World ACongress on Family Violence, held June 21-26, 2003, in Prague, Czech Republic.
  "Co-published simultaneously as Journal of elder abuse &neglect, volume 15, numbers 3/4, 2003." Includes bibliographical references and index.
      ISBN 0-7890-2823-9 (hard cover: alk. paper)–ISBN 0-7890-2824-7 (soft cover: alk. paper)
  1. Older people–Abuse of–Congresses. I. Podnieks, Elizabeth. II. Kosberg, Jordan I., 1939- III. Lowenstein, Ariela. IV. Journal of elder abuse & neglect. V. Title.
  HV6626.3.P73 2003
  362.6–dc22   205001520

Indexing, Abstracting & Website/Internet Coverage

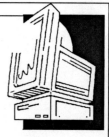

This section provides you with a list of major indexing & abstracting services and other tools for bibliographic access. That is to say, each service began covering this periodical during the year noted in the right column. Most Websites which are listed below have indicated that they will either post, disseminate, compile, archive, cite or alert their own Website users with research-based content from this work. (This list is as current as the copyright date of this publication.)

Abstracting, Website/Indexing Coverage . . . . Year When Coverage Began

- *Abstracts in Social Gerontology: Current Literature on Aging* **1991**
- *Academic ASAP <http://www.galegroup.com>* **1994**
- *Academic Search Elite (EBSCO)*. **1996**
- *Academic Search Premier (EBSCO)*
   <http://epnet.com/academic/acasearchprem.asp>. **1996**
- *AgeInfo CD-Rom <http://www.cpa.org.uk>* **1995**
- *AgeLine Database <http://research.aarp.org/ageline>* **1989**
- *Alzheimer's Disease Education & Referral Center*
   (ADEAR). **1995**
- *Behavioral Medicine Abstracts* **1992**
- *Business Source Corporate: coverage of nearly 3,350 quality*
   magazines and journals; designed to meet the diverse
   information needs of corporations; EBSCO Publishing;
   <http://www.epnet.com/corporate/bsourcecorp.asp> **1996**
- *CAB ABSTRACTS c/o CAB International/CAB ACCESS . . .*
   available in print, diskettes updated weekly, and on INTERNET.
   Providing full bibliographic listing, author affiliation, augmented
   keyword searching <http://www.cabi.org/> **2004**

(continued)

(continued)

(continued)

- *ProQuest 5000. Contents of this publication are indexed and abstracted in the ProQuest 5000 database (includes only abstracts . . . not full-text), available on ProQuest Information & Learning <http://www.proquest.com>* 1990
- *ProQuest Research Library. Contents of this publication are indexed and abstracted in the ProQuest Research Library database (includes only abstracts . . . not full text), available on ProQuest Information & Learning <http://www.proquest.com>* 1990
- *Psychological Abstracts (PsycInfo) <http://www.apa.org>* 2001
- *RESEARCH ALERT/ISI Alerting Services <http://www.isinet.com>* 2000
- *SafetyLit <http://www.safetylit.org>* 2004
- *Sage Family Studies Abstracts (SFSA)* 1995
- *Sage Urban Studies Abstracts (SUSA)* 1995
- *ScienceDirect Navigator (Elsevier) <http://www.info.sciencedirect.com>* 2002
- *Scopus (Elsevier) <http://www.info.sciencedirect.com>* 2002
- *Social Sciences Citation Index <http://www.isinet.com>* 1999
- *Social Scisearch <http://www.isinet.com>* 2000
- *Social Services Abstracts <http://www.csa.com>* 1990
- *Social Work Abstracts <http://www.silverplatter.com/catalog/swab.htm>* 1991
- *SocioAbs <http://www.csa.com>* 1990
- *Sociological Abstracts (SA) <http://www.csa.com>* 1990
- *SwetsWise<http://www.swets.com>* 2000
- *Violence and Abuse Abstracts: A Review of Current Literature on Interpersonal Violence (VAA)* 1995
- *Wilson Omnifile Full Text: Mega Edition (only available electronically) <http://www.hwwilson.com>* 1994

* Exact start date to come.

(continued)

Special Bibliographic Notes related to special journal issues (separates) and indexing/abstracting:

- indexing/abstracting services in this list will also cover material in any "separate" that is co-published simultaneously with Haworth's special thematic journal issue or DocuSerial. Indexing/abstracting usually covers material at the article/chapter level.
- monographic co-editions are intended for either non-subscribers or libraries which intend to purchase a second copy for their circulating collections.
- monographic co-editions are reported to all jobbers/wholesalers/approval plans. The source journal is listed as the "series" to assist the prevention of duplicate purchasing in the same manner utilized for books-in-series.
- to facilitate user/access services all indexing/abstracting services are encouraged to utilize the co-indexing entry note indicated at the bottom of the first page of each article/chapter/contribution.
- this is intended to assist a library user of any reference tool (whether print, electronic, online, or CD-ROM) to locate the monographic version if the library has purchased this version but not a subscription to the source journal.
- individual articles/chapters in any Haworth publication are also available through the Haworth Document Delivery Service (HDDS).

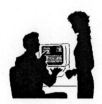

ABOUT THE EDITORS

Elizabeth Podnieks, EdD, RN, is Professor at Ryerson University, School of Nursing in Toronto and Chair of ONPEA. She conducted the National Survey on Abuse of the Elderly in Canada in 1991 and is a pioneer in elder abuse work in faith communities and raising awareness of elder abuse among children and adolescents. Dr. Podnieks has published extensively in the area of elder abuse and neglect, and has presented at numerous conferences, workshops, and scientific and educational meetings at both national and international levels. Included in the many conferences she has chaired and organized was the Second National Conference on Elder Abuse held in Toronto in 1999. She was the coordinator for Canada on the World Health Organization (WHO) International network for the Prevention of Elder Abuse (INPEA) global response to elder abuse, Vice-President of the INPEA, and a founding member of the Canadian Network for the Prevention of Elder Abuse (CNPEA). She was co-chair with Minister Cam Jackson on the Provincial Elder Abuse Round Table. Dr. Podnieks was awarded the Order of Canada for her work in the field of Elder Abuse in 2001.

Jordan I. Kosberg, PhD, ACSW, has been The University of Alabama Endowed Chair of Social Work since 1999. He has taught at numerous universities in the United States and has been a Visiting Professor at Nankai University in Tianjin, China, at Hong Kong University, at City University of Hong Kong, and was the 2002 Visiting TOWER Fellow of the New Zealand Institute for Research on Ageing at Victoria University of Wellington. He is a Fellow of The Gerontological Society of America (GSA) and of the Association for Gerontology in Higher Education (AGHE). Dr. Kosberg is editor or co-editor of six books, and author or co-author of 25 book chapters and over 100 journal articles. Dr. Kosberg is the Co-Principle Investigator for two research projects on family care giving funded by the National Institute on Aging and the Agency for Healthcare Research and Quality. He is former Board Member for the Association for Gerontology in Higher Education-Social Work (AGE-SW) and was awarded the Association's Career Achievement Award in 2000. He had been a member of the Board of Directors(representing the U.S.A. Region) for the International Network for the Prevention of Elder Abuse (a U.N. designated NGO).

Ariela Lowenstein, PhD, is Associate Professor and Head of the Department of Aging Studies-Master's in Gerontology, and the Center for Research and Study of Aging at the Faculty of Welfare and Health Studies, the University of Haifa, Israel. Dr. Lowenstein is considered one of the leading national and international experts in the field of aging. She has published extensively in several journals, chapters in books, monographs, and training manuals, and is co-editor of the books *Global Aging and the Family* and *The Need for Theory in Gerontology*. She serves as a research fellow at the Israeli Institute for Social Policy and the Herczg Institute for the Study of Aging at Tel-Aviv University, Israel, and also as an honorary fellow of the American Gerontological Society. She has extensive research collaboration with scholars from the U.S., Canada, and Europe and also serves on various Israeli governmental and local agencies as a consultant, member of various national committees and an advisor for policy planning. Dr. Lowenstein's research areas include intergenerational family relations, theory building in gerontology, grandparenthood, family care giving, elders' quality of life, elder abuse, gerontological education, policy development in aging, and service evaluation.

Elder Abuse: Selected Papers from the Prague World Conference on Family Violence

CONTENTS

Foreword

I am honored to have been invited to pen this foreword for the special collection entitled *Elder Abuse: Selected Papers from the Prague World Congress on Family Violence.*

Nothing that I might say can assuage the grief we have all felt at the loss of Gerry Bennett or the regret at the cancellation of the World Congress on Family Violence in Prague due to the "perfect storm" of international events–terrorism, SARS, and the Iraq war.

This special volume contains what would have been the presentations by a distinguished expert international faculty at the groundbreaking Elder Abuse Symposium in Prague, an international event dedicated to Gerry Bennett in recognition of his humanity, his spirit, and his leadership.

Those who had the privilege of knowing Gerry are aware of how much he cared about his work and his profession. His was a strong voice for the international effort to prevent family violence and especially elder abuse as General Secretary of the International Network for the Prevention of Elder Abuse (INPEA).

At the First World Conference on Family Violence in Singapore in 1998, I made a personal commitment to Gerry and to Rosalie Wolfe that elder abuse would be fully represented at any future World Congress. As Elizabeth Podnieks has written, "I greatly enjoyed the conference in Singapore but was concerned over the paucity of data on elder abuse." I believe Gerry felt that the commitment was kept. He played an active

---

[Haworth co-indexing entry note]: "Foreword." Davis, Alan. Co-published simultaneously in *Journal of Elder Abuse & Neglect* (The Haworth Maltreatment & Trauma Press, an imprint of The Haworth Press, Inc.) Vol. 15, No. 3/4, 2003, pp. xxi-xxii; and: *Elder Abuse: Selected Papers from the Prague World Congress on Family Violence* (ed: Elizabeth Podnieks, Jordan I. Kosberg, and Ariela Lowenstein) The Haworth Maltreatment & Trauma Press, an imprint of The Haworth Press, Inc., 2003, pp. xv-xvi. Single or multiple copies of this article are available for a fee from The Haworth Document Delivery Service [1-800-HAWORTH, 9:00 a.m. - 5:00 p.m. (EST). E-mail address: docdelivery@haworthpress.com].

xv

role as Honorary Co-Chair of the Second World Congress until his illness.

Gerry's beloved colleagues–Bridget Penhale, Silvia Perel Levins, Lia Daichman, and Elizabeth Podnieks among them–worked to prepare the Elder Abuse Symposium for the World Congress program during Gerry's illness and in his honor after his passing.

Special thanks to all of Gerry's colleagues and to members of the International Network for the Prevention of Elder Abuse (INPEA) for the substantial volunteer effort given to preparing the Symposium papers that appear in this special edition. I am grateful to them, to Terry Fulmer and to *JEAN* for this invaluable scholarly contribution to elder abuse literature.

The publication of the Prague Papers is a deserved salute to the growing international cadre of practitioners, researchers, and experts in the primary, secondary, and tertiary prevention of elder abuse for whom Gerry Bennett was in the vanguard.

Alan Davis
Chair of the International Steering Committee
World Congress on Family Violence (WCFV)
President and Chief Executive Officer
National Council on Child Abuse
and Family Violence (NCCAFV)
1025 Connecticut Avenue NW Suite 1012
Washington, DC 20036

Introduction

Elizabeth Podnieks, EdD, RN
Jordan I. Kosberg, PhD, ACSW
Ariela Lowenstein, PhD

The genesis of this volume has eloquently been expressed in the fore-word by Alan Davis. The "Prague Papers" is a bittersweet celebration of Gerry Bennett's contribution to the field of elder mistreatment. Of the eleven chapters, almost half are from international researchers. Gerry would have liked that. As editors, we would like to thank the contributors who have shared their ideas and insights in this volume.

Brownell, Berman, Nelson, and Fofana, have co-authored "Grand-parents Raising Grandchildren: The Risks of Caregiving," a report of the perceptions of grandparents and child welfare workers with regard to abusive behavior by grandchildren. Using a focus group methodology, the authors assess differences between the two groups in the perception of abusive (non-normative) and non-abusive (normative) behavior, and the existence–or lack–of needed services to preclude abuse by grandchildren. Differences were found between the two groups, as well as between African American and Latino grandparents. This research project has implications for the assessment of resources needed to assist in the prevention of abuse of grandparents by their grandchildren.

Also focusing upon the potential abuse of grandparents raising their grandchildren, Kosberg and MacNeil, in their article entitled "The El-

[Haworth co-indexing entry note]: "Introduction." Podnieks, Elizabeth, Jordan I. Kosberg, and Ariela Lowenstein. Co-published simultaneously in *Journal of Elder Abuse & Neglect* (The Haworth Maltreatment & Trauma Press, an imprint of The Haworth Press, Inc.) Vol. 15, No. 3/4, 2003, pp. 1-4; and: *Elder Abuse: Selected Papers from the Prague World Congress on Family Violence* (ed: Elizabeth Podnieks, Jordan I. Kosberg, and Ariela Lowenstein) The Haworth Maltreatment & Trauma Press, an imprint of The Haworth Press, Inc., 2003, pp. 1-4. Single or multiple copies of this article are available for a fee from The Haworth Document Delivery Service [1-800-HAWORTH, 9:00 a.m. - 5:00 p.m. (EST). E-mail address: docdelivery@haworthpress. com].

der Abuse of Custodial Grandparents: A Hidden Phenomenon," discuss the growth of such child care by "custodial grandparents" and their belief that abuse of these grandparents might be especially invisible. Using a Family Systems Perspective, the co-authors identify the dangerous combination of high-risk grandchildren and vulnerable grandparents. Grandparents are unlikely to admit to their abuse out of fear of the consequences to their grandchildren. Also discussed is the direct and indirect contribution of adult children to the abuse of custodial grandparents. The article concludes with a discussion of applied implications.

In their article, "Combating Elder Financial Abuse–A Multi-Disciplinary Approach to a Growing Problem," Malks, Buckmaster, and Cunningham discuss a model response, developed by the Financial Abuse Specialist Team (FAST), in Santa Clara County (California) to address financial abuse against older persons. A major goal of the program is the rapid response to freeze assets of older persons being financially abused before their resources are depleted. The authors conclude that FAST has been extremely successful in preventing incidents of economic abuse through early detection and the involvement of legal and law enforcement elements.

Kosberg, Lowenstein, Garcia, and Biggs, in their article "Study of Elder Abuse Within Diverse Cultures," present a discussion of the challenges for undertaking studies of cross-cultural and cross-national comparative analyses of elder abuse. The authors identify difficulties that result from varying definitions of elder abuse as a result of intra-country and cross-country differences, variations in methodologies used to study abuse, different measurement instruments, and a lack of a comprehensive theoretical framework that is ethnocentric "free."

Teaster, Nerenberg, and Stansbury present "A National Look at Elder Abuse Multidisciplinary Teams." Acknowledging the importance of such teams in a community's response to elder abuse, and with the assistance of the National Committee for the Prevention of Elder Abuse, the co-authors use a novel survey method to seek information from the coordinators from thirty-one such teams. Questions were asked about the process, structure, membership, leadership, funding, officers and terms of office, activities, and challenges. Among the findings from this descriptive survey is the importance of legal expertise to these teams. In addition to providing an overview of the functioning of such teams, the article can provide useful information for those from areas without such collaborative mechanisms by which to engage in elder abuse prevention, assessment, and intervention.

Koin, in her article "A Forensic Medical Examination Form for Improved Documentation and Prosecution of Elder Abuse," provides a description of a multidisciplinary assessment tool for the systematic documentation of information on abused persons as well as a procedure for describing the physical status of abuse victims. The developed tool emanated out of enabling California legislation that sought to improve reliable medical documentation for increased prosecution in abuse cases. The procedures and tools were created by a team of individuals from medicine, law enforcement, social services, and the legal profession, and for use by multi-disciplinary professionals. The article describes the need for training to use the form and the benefits of this formal protocol resulting in better identifying multiple patterns and forms of abuse and crimes, as well as providing baseline measures for intervention studies.

"Elder Abuse Awareness in Faith Communities: Findings from a Canadian Pilot Study," by Podnieks and Wilson, focuses upon the potentially important role of churches in the prevention of elder abuse. Religious leaders can be among the first group to encounter cases of abuse, yet they may be unaware of the possibility of abuse. Issues that are addressed by the faith leaders include the issue of confidential information received by congregants, the need for "sermonettes" for congregants regarding maltreatment of older persons, and the inclusion of gerontological material provided to students in schools of theology and seminaries. The co-authors conclude by advocating for the better preparation of those in the religious community.

Co-authors Podnieks and Wilson also reported in their article, "An Exploratory Study of Responses to Elder Abuse in Faith Communities" the results of a study on the perceptions of elder abuse by 49 religious leaders from many religious denominations in the Greater Toronto Area. These leaders were queried about their experiences with the problem of elder abuse among their congregants, the perception of barriers for disclosure by older persons and their families, and their responses to alleged or actual abuse. While it was found that the majority of religious leaders believe that they are aware that some elder abuse exists among their parishioners, they acknowledge a lack of knowledge about existing resources and interventions, and they see the need for more information and training.

Penhale is the author of "Older Women, Domestic Violence, and Elder Abuse: A Review of Commonalities, Differences, and Shared Approaches" in which she takes to task the lack of attention given to the interaction between abuse of older women and domestic violence. According to Penhale, older women may be considered to be especially vulnerable, dependent, and powerless. Although there are differences between the characteristics of domestic violence and elder abuse against females, there are commonalities related to the characteristics of the abuser, issue of empowerment, and policy and program interventions. Advocated is a feminist perspective that supports the idea that abuse of older women results, in part, on the basis of power inequities in society.

"Elder Abuse Risk Indicators and Screening Questions: Results from a Literature Search and a Panel of Experts from Developed and Developing Countries," is co-authored by Erlingsson, Carlson, and Saveman. Both the World Health Organization (WHO) and International Network for the Prevention of Elder Abuse (INPEA) have urged the development of a global detection instrument for elder abuse. Toward such an end, this article reports on a study that used a modified Delphi methodology and a literature search to arrive at consensus on risk indicators for elder abuse. A panel of 17 individuals representing different professional backgrounds from 12 developing and developed countries participated in the rank ordering of both risk indicators as well as screening items. The co-authors conclude that further work is needed before there can be common sets of criteria in the determination of elder abuse for global use and benefit.

It has been a great pleasure and privilege to work with the editor of *JEAN*, Dr. Terry Fulmer, and her associates Lisa Guadagno, and Marguarette Bolton-Blatt. Terry has guided and nurtured this volume from the beginning when she so enthusiastically accepted the concept of the "Prague Papers," right through to the completion and publication of the volume. Lisa and Marguarette, as associate editors, have shown infinite patience and flexibility in assisting the authors with revisions. We appreciate having had the unique opportunity to present this special collection of timely articles that we hope will be of interest to individuals working in the field of elder mistreatment, prevention, and treatment.

Grandparents Raising Grandchildren: The Risks of Caregiving

Patricia Brownell, PhD
Jacquelin Berman, PhD
Antoinette Nelson, MSSW, CSW
Rosemary Colon Fofana, MSW

SUMMARY. Findings from a study utilizing grandparent and child welfare worker focus groups demonstrate that professionals can learn about elder abuse from older people who may be experiencing abuse. This challenges the assumption that elder abuse is a social problem that must be defined by professionals because abuse victims are unable to speak for themselves. Differences in perceptions between African

---

Patricia Brownell is Assistant Professor, John A. Hartford Faculty Scholar, and Ravazżin Scholar, Fordham University Graduate School of Social Service, 113 West 60 Street, 7th Floor, New York, NY 10023 (E-mail: brownell@fordham.edu). Jacquelin Berman is Director of Research, New York City Department for the Aging, 2 Lafayette Street, New York, NY 10007 (E-mail: jberman@aging.nyc.gov). Antoinette Nelson is Director, Adoption Services, New York City Administration for Children's Services, 151 Williams Street, New York, NY (E-mail: 2335cs@acs.dfa. state.ny.us). Rosemary Colon Fofana is Social Worker, Municipal Employees Legal Services (MELS), District Council 37, 320 East 6th Street, #7, New York, NY 10003.

The authors would like to acknowledge the support of the Qualitative Research Work Group at the Fordham University Graduate School of Social Service.

[Haworth co-indexing entry note]: "Grandparents Raising Grandchildren: The Risks of Caregiving." Brownell, Patricia et al. Co-published simultaneously in *Journal of Elder Abuse & Neglect* (The Haworth Maltreatment & Trauma Press, an imprint of The Haworth Press, Inc.) Vol. 15, No. 3/4, 2003, pp. 5-31; and: *Elder Abuse: Selected Papers from the Prague World Congress on Family Violence* (ed: Elizabeth Podnieks, Jordan I. Kosberg, and Ariela Lowenstein) The Haworth Maltreatment & Trauma Press, an imprint of The Haworth Press, Inc., 2003, pp. 5-31. Single or multiple copies of this article are available for a fee from The Haworth Document Delivery Service [1-800-HAWORTH, 9:00 a.m. - 5:00 p.m. (EST). E-mail address: docdelivery@haworthpress.com].

http://www.haworthpress.com/web/JEAN
10.1300/J084v15n03_02

American and Latina grandparents underscore the importance of incorporating of diversity into elder abuse research. Examining elder abuse from the perspective of clients and professionals in service systems not traditionally associated with this social problem can promote case finding and prevention. *[Article copies available for a fee from The Haworth Document Delivery Service: 1-800-HAWORTH. E-mail address: <docdelivery @haworthpress.com> Website: <http://www.HaworthPress.com> © 2003 by The Haworth Press, Inc. All rights reserved.]*

KEYWORDS. Elder abuse, grandparents raising grandchildren, child welfare, aging, social services, intergenerational

INTRODUCTION

For most grandparents who care for grandchildren in the formal (child welfare) system or provide informal care, the kinship care arrangement represents opportunities to build a new family on a foundation of love, trust, familiarity, and commonality of culture. However, it can also mask family secrets, physical and psychological scars, deep disappointment and anger at the perceived failures of missing parents and children, and hope that the missing parents/children in the family will magically reappear (Holman, 2001). For older grandparents age 60 and above, it can bring added stress that exacerbates existing health conditions (Chalfie, 1994; Gilbert, 1998). It can mean other burdens for the custodial grandparents, including mistreatment by their own dependent grandchildren (Brownell & Berman, 2000).

To learn more about mistreatment of older custodial grandparents by grandchildren in their care, researchers from the Fordham University Graduate School of Social Service, the New York City Department for the Aging and the New York City Administration for Children's Services conducted an exploratory study of grandparents raising grandchildren and child welfare workers. The researchers conducted focus groups of grandparents raising grandchildren and child welfare workers to learn about their perceptions and experiences of mistreatment of grandparents by grandchildren in their care. The purpose was to identify and compare perceptions of grandparents raising grandchildren and child welfare workers on: (1) prevalence and types of grandchildren's behaviors toward grandparents associated with elder abuse; (2) available services that may be useful to grandparents coping with abusive grandchildren, and (3) services that may be useful but are not currently available. The study was funded by a Fordham University Faculty Research Grant.

KINSHIP CARE IN OLDER
GRANDPARENT-HEADED HOUSEHOLDS

The Census Bureau reports that nationwide, 2.4 million families in the United States are maintained by grandparents who have one more grandchildren living with them. This is an increase of 19 percent since 1990. Of the 4.5 million children under the age of 18 living in grandparent headed households, approximately two-thirds have no parent living in the household (U. S. Department of Commerce, 2003). Over one-third of families in kinship care live below the poverty line; of these families 76% have no earned income (Casper & Bryson, 1998). The majority of grandparents raising grandchildren are between the ages of 55 and 64; between 20-25 percent are over 65 years of age (AARP, 2004). A significant proportion of those are at least 60 years of age, defined by the Older Americans Act as the beginning of old age.

The term "kinship care" was first identified in work documenting the importance of kin networks in African American communities (Smith, 2000). Extended family and fictive kin (such as compadre or godparent) networks also have particular significance in the Latina culture (Hegar, 1999). Nationally, the prevalence of kinship care has increased over the past decade, especially in African-American and Latina families living in urban areas like New York City (Burnette, 1999). Children in kinship care are disproportionately African American, and children in public kinship care are more likely to be African American than children in non-kin foster care. Public kinship caregivers are also likely to be older, African American and experiencing economic and health difficulties (Chalfie, 1994; Gilbert, 1998; Han, 1995; U.S. Health and Human Services, 2000).

In spite of the economic disadvantages that many children in kinship foster care experience, studies of outcomes related to kinship foster care have found it to be beneficial to the overall family system. Children in kinship foster care have been found to be reunited with their parents more frequently than those in traditional foster care, move less often than in traditional care, and–for those who do leave the system–less likely to return to foster care (Courtney, White, & Klieman, 1997). Kinship care involving grandparents raising grandchildren in extended families has been particularly significant for African American families.

Although increasing numbers of kin are providing both formal and informal foster care for children, and the benefits of kinship care are well known in child welfare circles, little is done within that system to support and protect grandparents who are caring for troubled but beloved and needy grandchildren. According to administrators in the aging and child welfare fields, one reason for this is that too little is known about the risks faced by grandparents providing kinship care to children in the child welfare system, and few remedies short of removal are available to workers in the system (Brownell & Berman, 2000).

BACKGROUND

As the domestic violence service community became more involved with and concerned about abuse of older women, the view of elder abuse as a domestic violence issue began to transform the perception of elder abuse victims (Brandl, 2000). Earlier perceptions of impaired and care dependent elder abuse victims who, like children, could not be expected to speak out and advocate for themselves, evolved to include empowered older adult victims who could and should have a voice in the definition of their problems and the service solutions needed to address them. Understanding of abuser characteristics became more nuanced as well, suggesting the need to create new service models to supplement and complement those that emphasized supports for caregivers of victims as well as criminal prosecution of family perpetrators (Brownell, Berman, & Salamone, 1999). The work of Cox (2000) and Burnette (1999) has demonstrated the power and authority of grandparents who assume parenting roles for grandchildren if their grandchildren's parents are unable to undertake this responsibility. Grandparents raising grandchildren represent the category of empowered older adult victim of family mistreatment.

Child abuse and neglect has been identified as a social issue of concern since the 1960s, following the discovery of the battered children's syndrome (Kempe et al., 1962). By 1974, with the passage of the Child Abuse Prevention and Treatment Act (CAPTA) (P.L. 93-247), states began to establish child welfare systems for the reporting, detection, investigation, and protection of children who experienced or were at risk of harm by family members (Murray & Geririech, n.d.).

In contrast, elder abuse as a form of domestic violence was not identified as a serious social problem until the late 1970s (Wolf, 1988). The categories of behavior as directed toward a family member age 60 years or older that are defined as abuse or mistreatment include psychological abuse (threatening, yelling, name-calling, menacing, harming animals belonging to older person); financial (stealing money, taking possessions without the permission of the older adult), and physical (pushing, shoving, hitting) (Quinn & Tomita, 1997). Common to both conceptions of child abuse and elder abuse was the underlying assumption that both young and old victims of family abuse were care dependent and unable to speak effectively for themselves.

A review of the literature on abuse of grandparents by grandchildren shows passing references to dependent grandchildren listed among family abusers. This included a study on elder abuse and the criminal justice system (Brownell, 1998); a prevalence study conducted in Canada (Podnieks, 1992a and 1992b) and a study on abusers of elderly victims seeking assistance from the New York City Elderly Crime Victims Resource Center (Berman, 1998). These studies were conducted by gerontologists with older adults as subjects.

However, the issue of grandparents caring for abusive grandchildren has relevance for the child welfare system as well. The implementation of the Adoption and Safe Families Act (ASFA) of 1997 (P. L. 105-89) has raised concerns across the country about increasing numbers of permanency plans for pre-adoptive kinship families headed by grandparents with adolescent children that are failing. In response to ASFA, professionals working in the child welfare system are mandated to focus more attention than before the implementation of this legislation to achieving permanency for children removed from the care of abusive or neglectful parents. Preference is given to placing children with relatives, particularly grandparents, and if they are unable or unwilling to continue caring for these children, other less desirable arrangements must be made.

Research studies have documented abusive behaviors against older family members by sons and daughters (Anetzberger, 1987; Brownell, 1998; Steinmetz, 1988), and against older spouses (Pillemer & Finkelhor, 1989). However, there have been no studies published to date designed to focus specifically on similar behavior against custodial grandparents aged 60 years and older by their dependent grandchildren. While some studies have identified abuse of grandparents by dependent grandchildren (see Brownell, Berman, & Salamone, 1999; Brownell &

Berman, 2003), this study is the first to focus exclusively on abuse of custodial grandparents by dependent grandchildren in their care.

RESEARCH METHODOLOGY

Research Questions

Gerontologists may understand elder abuse as including physical, psychological and financial abuse; however, what does elder abuse mean to older adults caring for grandchildren, and child welfare who manage their cases in both the child welfare and public welfare systems. How do grandparents raising grandchildren, in contrast to the child welfare workers who serve them, define elder abuse? What are the services that grandparents raising grandchildren and their child welfare workers identify as helpful, and what services and supports are identified as needed but unavailable? Do grandparents differ in their perceptions of elder abuse and available and needed services differ based on their race/ethnicity?

First, the researchers were interested in understanding whether grandparents and child welfare workers considered mistreatment of grandparents by children–particularly adolescents–as prevalent, and if so, what specific behaviors they associated with mistreatment of grandparents by grandchildren, as compared with behaviors that could be considered abusive if perpetrated by an adult, but normative if perpetrated by a grandchild under the age of 18? Second, they were interested in learning whether grandparents and child welfare workers viewed available resources as helpful in addressing problems of abuse of grandparents by grandchildren. Third, they wanted to learn if there were resources and services that grandparents and child welfare workers thought could be useful but were unavailable at the present time.

The researchers felt it was important to know to whether grandparents and child welfare workers concurred or differed in the way they defined and categorized these behaviors. Also of significance was whether grandparents and child welfare workers concurred or differed on their assessment of available and needed resources; and what grandparents and child welfare workers identified as needed to prevent, detect and intervene in situations involving mistreatment of grandparents by grandchildren in their care.

Study Design

In order to learn more about older grandparents who are abused by grandchildren in their care, an exploratory study using focus groups was undertaken by researchers from the Fordham University Graduate School of Social Service, the New York City Department for the Aging and the New York City Administration for children's Services. According to the International Network for the Prevention of Elder Abuse (INPEA), "the focus group is becoming a popular qualitative research methodology used to elicit people's thoughts, attitudes, perceptions, and motives regarding social taboo topics, such as abuse and neglect of older adults" (INPEA, 2002, p.1). Another advantage of focus groups over individual interviews is that they foster intersubjectivity and generate responses through discussion: this has been found to be important in research on culturally taboo subjects like domestic violence (Yoshihama, 2002).

Data were collected through six focus groups: Three with older grandparents (60 years of age and older) caring for grandchildren, and three with child welfare caseworkers and supervisors who served grandparent-headed kinship foster care households on their caseloads. The focus groups were kept small (ranging from 8 to 12 participants) in order to facilitate active discussions. Funding and time constraints necessarily limited the numbers of focus groups included in the study; however, the researchers found that saturation was reached with subject topics after six focus group sessions were conducted: Three for grandparents and three for child welfare workers.

Participants

The grandparents who participated in the focus groups were recruited on a volunteer basis through grandparent support groups conducted under the auspices of the New York City Department for the Aging Grandparent Resource Center. The child welfare workers were recruited on a volunteer basis within the divisions of public and voluntary sector agencies that served kinship foster care cases. Child welfare worker focus groups were held during work hours. Care was taken to ensure that grandparents participating in focus groups were ethnically representative of kinship foster families in the New York City system. Two groups included primarily African-American and African-Caribbean grandparents, and one group was comprised solely of Hispanic grandmothers and conducted in Spanish. The ages of grandparents ranged from 61 through 80. All but one of the participating grandparents was female.

The child welfare workers participating in the focus groups represented a mix of African American, Latina, Caucasian, and African race/ethnic backgrounds. Two worker focus groups included direct care adoption and foster care workers from the public child welfare and one group consisted of workers from non-profit foster care agencies under contract with a public child welfare agency. Participating child welfare workers had at least a Bachelor's degree and several had Master's of Social Work degrees. The majority of child welfare workers who participated in the study were female.

While efforts were made to ensure participant ethnic and agency sector diversity in the participant selection process, the researchers did not select subjects randomly: subjects participated on a voluntary basis. As a result, the findings of the study cannot be generalized beyond the study sample; however, they have implications for practice, policy, and further research.

Session Procedures

All but one of the focus group discussions were facilitated by two professional social workers, with at least one graduate social work student taking notes. The Spanish-speaking focus group was facilitated by a Spanish-speaking social service worker and a Spanish-speaking retired nurse who received training in focus group methodology.

All participants volunteered and signed informed consent forms. The grandparents were each given gift certificates valued at $15.00 for their participation, in addition to travel expenses. Each group lasted two hours. Focus groups were conducted in 1999 and 2000. Grandparent focus groups were held at the New York City Department for the Aging, and two senior centers. The child welfare worker focus groups were held at the central public child welfare office. All subjects were assured that they could decide to discontinue participation in the research project without losing access to services or penalized in any way on the job. They were also told that all information was confidential, and that no names would be used in transcribing the audio-tapes or in the analysis of data.

Discussion question transcripts were utilized to structure and guide the focus group discussions. Participants were instructed that they did not have to divulge personal experiences if they chose not to, and could simply discuss what they heard from other grandparents. The grandparents were asked if they knew or heard of grandparents who they believed were mistreated by the grandchildren in their care and to discuss some ways that grandchildren behave that grandparents find annoying and some ways that grandchildren behave that are threatening or harmful. They were then asked to speak about some things that grandparents can do when grandchildren behave in threatening or harmful ways, and if grandparents reach out for assistance in these instances, where they can receive help. Finally, grandparents were asked to discuss what services they thought might be needed to provide more help, even if they did not exist now.

Child welfare workers were also asked if they knew or heard of grandparents who were mistreated by grandchildren in their care and what distinctions they would make among behaviors of adolescents toward grandparents they had observed or heard about that were annoying, and behaviors they identified as threatening or harmful They were asked about services they knew about that could be helpful to grandparents raising difficult grandchildren, and services that did not exist but were needed. Finally, they were asked to identify what services and supports would be helpful to them in working with grandparent-headed households.

Analysis

Focus groups were audiotaped, and audiotapes were transcribed. Transcripts were coded and analyzed using both manual methods and ATLIS.ti, a qualitative research software program. Focus groups are a type of group interview that utilizes a structured setting, a directive interviewer or facilitator, and a structured but open ended question format: The purpose is exploratory and designed to establish familiarity with a topic (Fontana & Frey, 2000).

Transcript analyses, as well as notes from focus group observers, were used to identify themes and compare responses between childcare workers and grandparents related to questions posed in the guided focus group discussions. Discussion questions were used as an organizing framework for a second round of data analysis, which used open and selective coding, and for presentation of data. While the Spanish-speaking focus group was transcribed and translated, the complexity of gaining meaning from Peruvian, Puerto-Rican, Bolivian, and Dominican speakers and translators required more reliance on notes taken during the session and from the audio-tape than in conducting a word by word analysis of the focus group transcript. Because the study used a purposive, non-random sample, findings cannot be generalized. However, findings can be used to generate ideas and implications for programs, policies and further research.

FINDINGS

Summary Theories

Grandparents and child welfare workers agreed that grandparents face unique challenges in raising older grandchildren. *Both groups concurred that grandparents do not always understand the contemporary social environment in which their grandchildren live;* they are conflicted about perceived failures with their children (parents of grandchildren in care); they sometimes lack the energy to keep up with the demands of raising grandchildren; and they chafe at the rules of the child welfare system, particularly in relation to corporal punishment and having young caseworkers tell them how to parent their grandchildren. Grandparents identified harmful behaviors of grandchildren toward grandparents as a significant risk for kinship caregiving in both formal and informal child care systems. Child welfare workers, in contrast, did not perceive this as significant although they recognized that they were not trained to recognize it, and acknowledged that it may be more prevalent than they realized.

Both child welfare workers and grandparents concurred on the behaviors they identified as physically harmful to grandparents. The two groups differed, however, on the perception of prevalence of this category of abuse in kinship foster home settings. According to grandparents participating in the focus groups, physical abuse of grandparents by grandchildren is not uncommon, only hidden, because there is an incentive to conceal this from their child welfare workers. Child welfare workers, predictably, reported that they rarely witness or hear of it, and expressed skepticism that it existed.

Both grandparents and child welfare workers categorized harmful or abusive behaviors in ways similar to gerontologists: As physically, financially, and psychologically abusive. However, neither group identified neglect of grandparents as a category of harmful or abusive behavior demonstrated by grandchildren. This is not surprising as grandparents are assumed to be caregivers of dependent children by the child welfare system. However, grandparents identified a fourth category: That of disrespectful behavior. They identified behaviors associated with this category as verbal or nonverbal behavior, disobedient behavior, and low-level financial abuse. Workers rarely identified this as a category of behavior and then only to question whether it was distinct from normal difficult child and adolescent behavior. In addition, African-American and Latina grandparents classified different behaviors as disrespectful. African-American grandparents were more likely to classify behaviors such as disobeying curfew, being truant from school, or talking back as disrespectful, while Latina grandparents identified forms of non-verbal behavior like refusing to respond to questions or making faces as disrespectful.

Child welfare workers and grandparents also differed in their perception of financial abuse, as defined by gerontologists. Child welfare workers were ambivalent about defining stealing as a form of abusive behavior. While not condoning it, child welfare focus group participants identified stealing as so prevalent as to be relatively normative. Grandparents distinguished between stealing small amounts of money or non-valuable possessions, which they categorized as disrespectful behavior, and stealing large amounts of money and valuables, which they categorized as abusive.

Finally, child welfare workers and grandparents differed as to what behaviors they defined as psychological, including verbal, abuse. Child welfare workers were more likely to define behaviors like cursing, school truancy, and disobeying curfews set by grandparents as unpleasant but normative adolescent behavior, reflecting testing of boundaries and beginning the separation and individuation process. Grandparents, on the other hand, were more likely to define these behaviors as disrespectful. Grandparents also expressed concern that if not addressed, what they defined as disrespectful behavior could escalate into abusive behavior.

Grandparents and child welfare workers concurred with one another on identification of the services they felt were available and useful, as well as those they felt were unavailable but needed. Grandparents identified both informal and formal sources of support as important to their responsibilities as kinship parents for grandchildren, while child welfare workers focused on elements of the formal service system. Child welfare workers stated that if they were to learn more about existing services for grandparents raising grandchildren, they could be more effective in providing assistance to grandparents by identifying and linking them to these services. Child welfare workers also expressed interest in advocating on behalf of grandparents for needed, but currently unavailable, services.

Identifying and Categorizing Abusive Behaviors

Grandparents made a distinction between what they defined as annoying but normative adolescent behavior, what they defined as disrespectful behavior, and what they defined as threatening or harmful behavior. Although facilitators did not use the word "abuse" or the phrase "elder abuse," grandparents did on several occasions use these terms to describe threatening behavior by grandchildren toward grandparents.

Child welfare workers, many with Master's of Social Work degrees, reflected an exposure to theories of child and adolescent development stages. They were more likely to identify as normal or annoying those categories of adolescent behavior that grandparents had identified as disrespectful or threatening. Child welfare workers categorized many adolescent behaviors differently than the grandparents. Refusing to attend school and respect curfews were more likely to be seen by the workers as part of normal adolescent testing of boundaries and beginning the separation and individuation tasks of adolescence. Grandparents also recognized that adolescence was a stage in a child's life when rebellion may take the form of challenging authority or not completing assigned household chores. However, they felt that some behaviors, while not threatening or harmful to the grandparent, showed disrespect.

These included behaviors like cursing, talking back to the grandparent, disobeying curfews set by the grandparent, and truancy at school. Grandparents defined as disrespectful stealing small amounts or non-valuable possessions of the grandparent. Failure to heed requests was also described by grandparents as disrespectful: "Every night he be playing that music all night, that television will be on all night. When I go and just get up and say please turn it off, and he would turn it down and as soon as I go back in the room, it's on again . . . up to last night, up to last night. " "He won't listen to me and if his father come to the house and say, 'Take that off!,' " "It's off." "He don't listen to me." "They don't want to obey us." Lying was another behavior that grandparents identified as disrespectful: "To me, it is very annoying when you look at a child and you see what they is doing and they turn right around and say they didn't do it." Another said: "You tell them to do something and they got some words to say; they talk back."

Grandparents identified as abusive behaviors such as punching, hitting, throwing objects, stealing money that was needed for the household or stealing prized possessions, destroying possessions, and threatening the grandparent with weapons. One grandparent stated: "Yeah, they steal from out of the house, take things out of the house, that you know, well, when you've been somewhere for 40 years, you accumulate a lot of stuff and a lot of it you recognize but you don't know where you have it. So I see these things, she'll bring it back in and she'll say, 'Oh, my friend gave it to me.'"

Etiology of Identified Abusive Behavior

Some grandparents indicated that they felt the underlying motivation of the behavior was a mitigating factor in whether behavior should be considered disrespectful, as opposed to threatening or abusive. One grandparent stated that her granddaughter's behavior became much worse after she had contact with her mother, who was a substance abuser and had neglected her daughter. As another grandparent noted: "Some things grandchildren do, they need help. They need psychology. They need to go to a therapist. Doctors. And let them see if they can find out what the child needs."

Workers expressed concern that grandparents faced unique challenges in raising older grandchildren and believed that the grandparents did not always understand the contemporary environment in which their grandchildren were living. They felt that the grandparents were conflicted about their own perceived failures with the parents of the grandchildren in their care (their own children), and that they sometimes lacked the energy to keep up with the demands of raising grandchildren, and may neglect their own health needs to keep the myriad of appointments required of the foster care system. Child welfare workers acknowledged that the grandparents chafe against the rules of the agency in relation to corporal punishment and having young caseworkers telling them how to raise their grandchildren. As one participant stated: "They've done their parenting, and this is the second time around. It's very hard for a lot of them, and it's very hard for [child welfare workers] to come in and tell them 'This is what you have to do' when they figure they have already raised their children. Most of them don't really know what happened with their own daughter. They say they raised her the best that they could."

Psychological or Verbal Abuse

Grandparents viewed psychological or verbal abuse by grandchildren as disrespectful and a precursor to more harmful behavior. Grandparents firmly stated that unless disrespectful behavior such as talking back to a grandparent was addressed early on, the grandchild's behavior was likely to escalate to more abusive actions. They chafed against the constraints imposed by the family court and child welfare agency against corporal punishment, which they believed severely limited their options for disciplining grandchildren and preventing escalation of disrespectful and abusive behavior by grandchildren. As one grandmother stated: "And then you can't do anything, you can't hit them, you can't chastise them, you can't punish them. You can't do it, and they like . . . hum! You know."

Child welfare workers identified cursing and talking back to grandparents as annoying as opposed to abusive behavior, and acknowledged difficulty in distinguishing verbal "dissing" (or disrespectful behavior) from unpleasant but normative adolescent behavior. One participant stated: "I am struggling with this disrespectful thing. . . . Two things are going on. You're asking an adolescent who at this time of their life needs to separate from authority. We'll look at any normal teenager at home and they'll say 'parent, you're stupid, you know nothing.' I've had that with my own children. My issue is how much of that behavior is normal and how much of this behavior does the grandparent know is normal? Are we asking this child to do something contrary to developmental issues?"

Financial/Material Abuse

Stealing money needed for household expenses, or destroying or stealing valued possessions were examples of behaviors that grandparents identified as financially abusive. Comments include: "Sometimes they steal all the money, like taking the check at the beginning of the month and then you can't pay your rent and other bills." "One child stole from the grandparent and the grandparent didn't know how much she had taken. But then she kept stealing five dollars here and five dollars there and pretty soon it was $40.00." Latina grandparents were less likely to view stealing as abusive, compared with African American grandparents. To Latina grandparents, it was viewed as a moral issue.

Unlike grandparents who identified stealing small sums of money as disrespectful and large sums of money or valuables as abusive, child welfare workers viewed stealing from grandparents as normative. While not condoning this and recognizing the hardships it created for grandparents living and raising grandchildren on fixed incomes, they stated that stealing was extremely common and occurred in most kinship foster care households. On the other hand, workers made a link between financial, verbal, and physical abuse: "Verbal abuse over money generally leads to physical abuse," one participant stated.

Physical Abuse

Grandparents identified aggressive physical behavior of grandchildren toward grandparents as abusive, but generally ascribed a psychological or psychiatric motive for it. One grandparent stated: "Some are physically abusive. They punch, beat, throw things, swear, hit. It's anger. They don't know how to cope with it." Another said: "You get these kids that's under this medication, they get out of control, they beat anybody that is in their sight." A third grandparent said: "I have a friend. Her granddaughter is 13-years-old and . . . she went out to a party last week, week before last. She told the child to be home at 10:00 and the child didn't come home until 1:00 and when the grandparent was asking her questions she took a chair and hit her grandmother in the head. She's in the hospital now." "Well, if they physically abuse you, that's threatening because they can hurt you. And some kids do throw weapons, they throw at their grandparents. And, even their parents, but much more their grandparents." Grandparents stated that physical abuse was in fact common, but they concealed it from their child welfare workers to protect their grandchildren against removal.

Child welfare workers insisted that physical abuse was extremely rare, although they acknowledged that grandparents sometimes conceal physical abuse out of shame or to protect against the removal of the abusive child and his or her siblings. According to one worker, "I had a 14-year-old boy [on my caseload] who was 6'2" and 180 pounds and he was abusing his grandmother and she would never tell. She kept coming up with excuses that she had these accidents, broken legs, broken arms, broken ribs. It was always that she fell down the stairs even though she never took anything but the elevator!" However, another participant, when asked what proportion of cases he knew or heard about that was abusive as compared with disrespectful, responded: "Maybe 10 percent is abusive." Asked to define the frequency of physical abuse, as compared with financial or psychological abuse, the participant stated: "Less frequent for me." Another worker stated: "Based on what we hear at [case] conferences, hitting is not really an issue; it is more of an exception."

Use of Services

Grandparents and child welfare workers identified many of the same services identified as useful and available, although unlike the grandparents child welfare workers focused primarily on the availability of and need for supports in the formal service system. Child welfare workers also felt that they did not know enough about services for grandparents. As one worker stated: "Speaking as a caseworker, I primarily know resources for children and for the birth parents. Unfortunately, I'm going to be honest, I don't really know that many resources for the grandparent."

Counseling

Both grandparents and child welfare workers identified counseling as helpful for both grandparents and grandchildren. As one grandparent stated: " I think the main thing is counseling. Even before a grandchild gets sent out, I feel they should have counseling, like everyone here said, to know how to deal with this form of behavior. To let them know that these are some of the things that you are going to expect, and this is how you should deal with it. And if you find yourself with a problem, you can give them phone numbers that they can have and have emergency meetings, or whatever." Some grandparents received professional counseling through a clinic or faith community, and identified this as a useful support. Although one grandmother said: "When the child has a counselor, they have to deal with you as well." Child welfare workers identified counseling as an important service for both grandchildren and grandparents, both for prevention and intervention purposes.

Faith-Based Services

Grandparents identified their faith and the support of their church as a key support for them. As one grandparent put it: "If I had a problem I would definitely call the church." Another said: "I just pray to God constantly."

Child welfare workers also identified faith-based social services, such as social services, scouting and mentoring with male role models as important supports for grandparents raising grandchildren. One worker said: "The grandparents, a lot of them are very resourceful. I know a lot of mine are spiritual people." Unlike the grandparents, however, they believed that these supports already existed.

Grandparent Support Group Members

For those attending the focus groups organized with assistance by the New York City Department for the Aging Grandparent Resource Center, grandparent support groups were identified as helpful. Focus group members noted, however, that some grandparents they knew who were experiencing abuse by grandchildren in their care refused to come to support group meetings in spite of invitations to attend by support group members (Grandparent Resource Center, n.d.). Child welfare workers stated that they were unaware that grandparent support groups existed, but thought they could be helpful to grandparents on their caseloads.

Schools

Grandparents noted appreciation for the support of personnel in their grandchildren's schools. While guidance counselors were singled out for praise by African American grandparents, Latina grandparents identified their grandchildren's teachers as helpful.

Child welfare workers stated they believed that opportunities for adolescents in kinship foster care to come together to discuss common issues and concerns could ease tensions in grandparent-headed households. They identified the schools as providing these support groups, but also suggested that the child welfare system could take some responsibility for establishing groups like this also.

Case Conferencing

While grandparents did not mention case conferences as useful services, child welfare workers expressed concern over the multiple systems, including health, education and social services, grandparents had to negotiate to maintain grandchildren in their custody. Child welfare workers felt that they were able to more effectively support grandparents who were raising adolescent grandchildren through case conferencing with professionals in these systems.

Formal services that grandparents, but not caseworkers, identified as important for them included community hospitals, police, elected officials, and the child welfare system itself. Grandparents felt they could utilize community hospitals for assistance with extreme cases of abuse or when grandchildren showed symptoms of physical or psychiatric disorders that may have contributed to the abusive behaviors.

Police

Grandparents looked to local police to assist them in enforcing authority over grandchildren, particularly those who were engaging in disrespectful behavior. The police were also viewed as role models for adolescent boys in their care, and the police appeared to be willing to assume this role if called to a household by a grandmother struggling with disciplining an adolescent boy. As one stated: [when the policeman came in response to a call regarding a problem with grandsons] "and he told them you are in a good home, you have your family." Participants also thought police could help more than they did, however. Responding to a question regarding the police response to a call regarding an abusive grandchild, one participated noted: "There's very little the police does. They'll take them from the house and they'll drop them not so far away and then you look and they're back again. I think it's best to go through a program like you say."

Local Elected Officials

Latina grandparents, but not African American grandparents, identified local elected officials as helpful in assisting them with grandchildren's problems.

Child Welfare Workers

Finally, in spite of concern about the potential that child welfare workers had for exerting unwanted authority over them and their relationships with their grandchildren, many grandparents expressed appreciation for the support and encouragement they received from their caseworkers. One participant observed, when asked about services grandparents could seek if they were having problems with their grandchildren: "You call, first you talk to your agency, your worker."

Grandparents, but not child welfare workers, also identified informal support systems like family and friends as providing important services to them. Family, including fictive kin, and friends provided social network support: Male relatives such as uncles, if available, were identified as important for mentoring adolescents in their care. One grandparent stated: "I find calling a friend, a few friends, with what the

few say to you can help out a lot." Another grandparent, who was raising two grandsons, said: "They always had a trusted friend that they
would call uncle and a lot of times I would tell them Uncle Mike want
you and then a lot of time Uncle Mike would take them out or let them
come in and talk to them and then relieve the problem."

However, they noted the vulnerabilities of relying on family and
friends as well. One participant recollected: "That brings me back to
something a grandparent had mentioned that they were raising a grandchild and she was being very [disrespectful] so they ask a friend, a male
friend, to talk to her. The male friend ended up abusing the granddaughter . . ."

Service Needs

Both grandparents and child welfare workers identified a number of
service needs that needed to be addressed by the formal service system.
These included respite services for grandparents and grandchildren,
greater recognition of grandparents raising grandchildren, and psychiatric services for troubled grandchildren.

Grandparents believed they could benefit from occasional time away
from their grandchildren. Because of lack of sufficient economic and
social support resources, they suggested that a formal program providing in-home supervision of grandchildren and an occasional weekend
trip for grandparents would be helpful. One grandmother suggested: "I
got two things I think would work out. If I had a wish, I would wish that
they would have a grandparents' house . . . yeah, a special place to go
temporarily."

Grandparents also felt that structured opportunities for grandchildren
to spend time away from the household, such as overnight camps, could
provide relief for grandparents. As one grandparent put it: " I know certain organizations have camps for children, but we have no camps for
grandparents' children. Camps just for grandparents' children. Yes, uh
huh, I think that would be nice. Then grandparents would know they
would get at least one week of rest and the kids would be taken care of."

More Recognition of Service

Grandparents felt that if there was more public recognition of their
efforts to care for their grandchildren, their morale would be boosted
and their grandchildren would respect them more. They suggested that

public officials designate an official Grandparent's Day and hold annual recognition ceremonies. As one grandparent noted: "We know that grandparents have been doing this for years and years now haven't got the recognition for it. And this age now, they need to be brought up that they are individuals, they are people too, they need to be recognized for what they are doing." Another grandparent discussed the stigma grandchildren felt being raised by grandparents instead of their parents: "So it's like, you know, I don't know, they kind of was ashamed because kids was all, oh, your grandparents is raising you, and they won't tell nobody that their grandparents are raising them because children do make fun of them." "Yeah. Yeah. You don't have no parents because your grandparents is raising you and they won't tell anyone who is raising them. They say, 'I live with my grandparents.' They will say 'I LIVE,' but they will not say that their grandparents are raising them."

Child welfare workers concurred with the grandparents that more could be done to recognize grandparents for the services they provide. One worker stated: "We could do it for the [kinship] foster grandparents. They should be rewarded . . . It's hard, it's very hard to keep doing it."

Grandparent Training and Orientations

Both grandparents and child welfare workers recognized the need for grandparents to obtain more training and orientation on raising grandchildren, particularly those who had traumatic experiences prior to joining their household. Grandparent orientation upon assuming role of kinship foster parent: Child welfare workers expressed concern that grandparents often assumed responsibility for grandchildren during crises that precipitated emergency removal from biological parents, and were not provided an opportunity to learn what was expected of them as kinship foster parents prior to making the commitment to care for their grandchildren. They concurred with grandparents that this was not made available to grandparents in a timely way.

One grandparent stated: "What she was saying is that, the training, but you are calling to take these kids, there is no training. They say, 'Look, come and get your grandkids otherwise we be putting them in foster care.' Somehow you afraid to say anything to anyone because they may take the kids from you until you get that training. So, a lot of grandparents don't say anything, they just take their grandchildren and do the best they can." Grandparents identified an interest and need to learn more about the dynamics of domestic violence as they related to intergenerational relationships between dependent grandchildren and grandparents. They complained that traditional domestic violence programs were not relevant to their situations.

Specialized Services for Disturbed Grandchildren

Both grandparents and child welfare workers identified a need for additional services for severely disturbed grandchildren in the child welfare system. Child welfare workers acknowledged that more needed to be done proactively to address emerging problems with troublesome grandchildren before their behavior escalated to abuse. They identified counseling as needed to be provided in the early stages of grandchild-grandparent conflict.

Child welfare workers concurred with grandparents that specialized services were needed for grandchildren with severe psychiatric problems. They recommended that all children coming into care, but particularly those who had experienced severe abuse or neglect, be given comprehensive neurological examinations to detect problems and assist grandparents in dealing with these problems. Grandparents identified grandchildren's substance abuse and mental illness as two factors related to abusive behavior toward grandparents. They expressed concern that there should be specialized services available and provided to disturbed and abusive adolescents before consideration of removal from grandparents' households by the child welfare system.

Grandparents and child welfare workers also differed in the service gaps they identified in the focus groups. While grandparents listed community hospitals as providing important services for them and their grandchildren, they also identified gaps in the community based health care system. According to one grandparent; " . . . there will come a time, when we are not going to be well all the time and this way, if someone was there, you know, we all combine with the grandchildren what not, and they have doctors' appointments. If the grandparents be sick, they will be going to the hospital, the doctors will be right there to help us. Cause we need a hand every now and then."

Some cultural differences emerged in the discussion of service gaps for grandparent headed households. Latina but not African American grandparents identified a need for court-based mandated services that would force problematic grandchildren to assume personal responsibility for their actions. Apparently the Latina grandparents felt that only a court-mandated process was going to force a grandchild into a program.

Grandparents identified their faith communities as important supports in their lives, and suggested that more services for themselves and their grandchildren should be based in their churches. They also identified male faith community leaders and members as important role models for their male grandchildren. Grandparents acknowledged that they were raising their grandchildren in a different world from the one in which they had grown up or the one in which they had raised their children. They sought ways to identify opportunities for bridging cultural gaps with their grandchildren by participating in activities that would bring them closer to their grandchildren's world.

Finally, grandparents felt frustrated that their grandchildren were not provided with information on what the child welfare system required of grandparents and particularly that the purpose of the foster care stipend was to maintain a household for grandchildren and grandparent. They complained that some adolescents demanded that the stipend be given to them directly, accusing the grandparent of withholding funds that belonged to them for their personal use. One grandparent observed: "That's the hard part about raising your grandchild. Because our pension is not that great because during our time, they didn't pay that much money. So your old pension is not that great. So you have expenses, any house expenses."

Child welfare workers, on the other hand, wanted more training in gerontology and services that are available to older adults in their communities. They recognized that they were in a position to address service gaps for the grandparents raising grandchildren on their caseloads, and wanted the professional knowledge and skills to do so more effectively.

The child welfare workers participating in the focus groups observed that there were increasing numbers of older grandparents raising grandchildren in the kinship foster care program; however, the workers felt unprepared to provide adequate support for these grandparents. They stated that they would welcome training to help them understand the issues of adults in later life, as well as services available to grandparents and older adults through the aging service system. As one worker stated: " Now, when you say training, originally I thought training for the grandparent but the training would also be beneficial for the agency workers" Another said: "So they do need, all the way around something that, you know, that's always going to be there because like I said, I don't think the population of children being placed with relatives, with grandparents, is going to decrease. There's always a new drug out there, there's always more problems in society . . ."

Child welfare workers were also unaware of many services available to grandparents in the aging service system, including grandparent support groups. They identified a need for grandparent support groups, not realizing that they already existed. One worker observed: "This goes along with peer counseling for the teens. The grandparents may also be able to have the same thing because if you're a new grandparent that's now a foster parent, who better to learn from than some of them that have been doing it already."

Cultural Influences

As noted, some differences in perceptions of annoying but normal, disrespectful, and abusive behaviors of grandchildren in their care emerged between the African American and Latina grandparents. Latina grandparents expressed more nuanced concern about non-verbal behaviors on the part of their grandchildren, which they tended to experience as disrespectful and abusive, and to which they assigned a moral value. They also expressed more respect for and reliance on teachers and law enforcement than did the African American grandparents. It was the Latina grandparents who suggested that local elected officials could be helpful to grandparents in solving problems with their grandchildren. African American grandparents expressed concern about restrictions on corporal punishment in the kinship foster care program, which they felt limited the authority they could exert over their grandchildren, and chafed against the oversight provided by the child welfare system.

The importance of understanding elder abuse from a cultural perspective is recognized by the elder abuse research community (Tatara, 1999). Studies on elder abuse among Japanese Americans, American Indians, Latinas, Asian Americans, and African Americans have begun to expand our understanding of elder abuse in these communities, in spite of small samples and limited access. Considering each culture's definition of elder abuse has been identified as essential, including those cultures that value the community over individual needs (Rittman, Kuzmeskus, & Flum, 1999).

Implications for Social Work Practice and Policy

Relatives are generally expected to provide support as well as resources in a family crisis. Family support is a crucial survival mechanism for many families. Families in crisis, in most instances depend on the grandparent for a variety of financial and emotional support. In Black and Latina families, grandparents often occupy a central position in the family network, particularly for children living in chaotic and unstable conditions. Substance abusing parents, teen mothers, parents who have been incarcerated, and those with chronic physical or mental illness may depend on grandparents as substitute caregivers. Minority grandparents often make tremendous sacrifices to care for grandchildren maltreated by their overly dependent adult children.

Both grandparents and child welfare workers identified a need for more existing services for both grandparents and grandchildren in the kinship foster care system. They also expressed a need for services that did not exist, such as community-based one stop clinics and service programs that both grandparents and grandchildren could utilize.

Child welfare workers in particular recommended that there be more collaboration and information sharing between the child welfare and aging service systems to enable them to support grandparents raising grandchildren more effectively. Another outcome of the study for the researchers is the recognition that a new paradigm of elder abuse is needed, incorporating dimensions of child welfare and grandparent caregiving. One elder abuse myth is that all victims are frail and care dependent (Prichard, 1993). First, this inhibits case finding and development of new and successful interventions. Second, it is challenged by the reality of strong and vital grandparents who raise grandchildren against great odds, and who can be considered "heros of their own lives" (Gordon, 1988).

Finally, study findings demonstrate that grandparents have a great deal to say about issues related to the kinship foster care system, and what is needed to address them. It is essential for social workers to work collaboratively with grandparents. It is also essential for policymakers to include grandparents and gerontological experts in drafting intergenerational child welfare policy that addresses the unique needs of elderly caregivers.

Implications for Further Research

Findings from grandparent and child welfare worker focus groups demonstrated that clients can differ from professionals about definitions of social problems and strategies for addressing them. Elder abuse is an example of a social problem that was defined by professionals with the underlying assumption that the victims were unable to speak for themselves. The perceptions of elder abuse, the behaviors associated with it, and the services needed to address it, as articulated by the grandparents in the study, challenge the notion that professionals cannot learn about elder abuse from older people who may experience it. Differences in perceptions between the African American and Latina grandparents reinforce the importance of incorporating considerations of diversity into elder abuse research (Tatara, 1999). Examining elder abuse from the perspective of clients and professionals in service systems not traditionally associated with this social problem can expand our understanding of it and ensure that hidden cases of elder abuse are identified and addressed (Brownell, Welty, and Brennan, 2000). Finally, it is important to take into consideration the needs of elder abuse perpetrators like minor grandchildren who themselves may be incapable of fully understanding the consequences of their behavior and who have unique service needs of their own.

REFERENCES

Anetzberger, G. (1987). The etiology of elder abuse by adult offspring. Springfield, IL: Charles C. Thomas.

Berman, J. (1998). Preliminary report on senior crime victims and grandparent abuse. New York: Department for the Aging.

Brandl, B. (2000). *Power and control: Understanding domestic abuse in later life.* Generations, xxiv, 11, 39-41.

Brownell, P. (1998). *Family crimes against the elderly: Elder abuse and the criminal justice system.* New York: Garland Publishing Company.

Brownell, P., and Berman, J. (2000). Risks of caregiving: Abuse within the relationship. In Cox, C. B. (Ed.), *To grandmother's house we go . . . and stay: Perspectives on custodial grandparents.* New York: Springer Publishing Company, 91-109.

Brownell, P., and Berman, J. (2003). Elder abuse femicides. In Roberts, A. R., and Greene (Eds.), *Handbook of Evidence-based Practice.* New York: Oxford University Press.

Brownell, P., Berman, J., and Salamone, A. (1999). Mental health and criminal justice issues among perpetrators of elder abuse. *Journal of Elder Abuse & Neglect,* 1, 4, 1999, 81- 93.

Brownell, P., Welty, A., and Brennan, M. (2000). Elder abuse and neglect. *In Project 2015: The Future of Aging in New York State, Articles for Discussion.* Albany, NY: New York State Office for the Aging.

Burnette, D. (1999). Custodial grandparents in Latino families: Patterns of service use and predictors of unmet needs. *Social Work,* 44, 1, 22-34.

Casper, L. M., and Bryson, K. R. (1998). *Co-resident grandparents and their grand-children: Grandparent maintained households.* Washington, DC: U. S. Bureau of the Census. Population Division Working Paper No. 26.

Chalfie, D. (1994, September). *Going it alone: A closer look at grandparents parenting children.* Washington, DC: American Association of Retired Persons.

Charmaz, K. (2000). Grounded theory: Objectivist and constructivist methods. In Denzin, N. K., and Lincoln, Y. S. (Eds.), *Handbook of qualitative research methods, 2nd edition).* Thousand Oaks, CA: Sage, 509-535.

Courtney, J., White, A., & Keliman, V. S. (Eds.). (Spring 1997). *Child Welfare Watch.* New York City: Center for an Urban Future and the New York Forum.

Cox, C. (Ed.). (2000). *To grandmother's house we go . . . and stay: Perspectives on custodial grandparents.* New York: Springer Publishing Company, 91-109.

Erikson, E. H. (1997). The life cycle completed. New York: W. W. Norton & Company.

Fontana, A., and Frey, J. H. (2000). The interview: From structured questions to negotiated text. In Denzin, N. K., and Lincoln, Y. S. (Eds.), *Handbook of Qualitative Research, Second Edition.* Thousand Oaks, CA: Sage Publications, 645-672.

Fromm, E. (1964). The heart of man. New York: Harper & Row.

Gilbert, S. (July 28, 1998). *Rising stress of raising a grandchild.* The New York Times, F7.

Gordon, L. (1988). *Heroes of their own lives the politics and history of family violence.* New York: Viking.

Grandparent Resource Center (n.d.). A *helping hand for grandparents who are raising grandchildren.* New York: Department for the Aging.

Han, S. (March 19, 1995). *Grandma, what big worries you have.* Daily News, 5.

Hegar, R. L. (1999). The cultural roots of kinship care. In Hegar, R. L., & Scannapieco, M. (Eds.), *Kinship foster care: Policy, practice, and research.* New York: Oxford University Press, 17-27.

Holman, D. (2001). Reaching for integrity: An Eriksonian life-cycle perspective on the experience of adolescents being raised by grandparents. *Child and Adolescent Social Work Journal,* 21-34.

International Network for the Prevention of Elder Abuse (2002). Listening to the missing voices. Views on elder abuse: A focus group approach. Geneva, Switzerland: World Health Organization.

Kempt, C. H., Silverman, F. N., Steele, B. F., Droegemuller, W., and Silver, H. K. (1992). *The battered child syndrome.* Journal of the American Medical Association, 181, 17-24.

Murray, K. O., and Gesiriech, S. (n.d.). A *brief legislative history of the child welfare system.* (*http://pewfostercare.org*)

Pillemer, K., and Finkelhor, D. (1989). Causes of elder abuse: Caregiver stress versus problem relatives. *American Journal of Orthopsychiatrist, 59* (2), 179-187.

Podnieks, E. (1992a). Emerging themes from a follow-up study of Canadian victims of elder abuse. *Journal of Elder Abuse & Neglect* 4 (1/2), 59-111.

Podnieks, E. (1992b). National survey on abuse of the elderly in Canada. *Journal of Elder Abuse & Neglect 4*(1/2), 5-58.

Prichard, J. (1993). Dispelling some myths. *Journal of Elder Abuse & Neglect, 5*(2), 27-37.

Quinn, M. J., & Tomita, S. K. 1997). *Elder abuse and neglect: Causes, diagnosis, and intervention strategies, Second edition.* New York: Springer Press.

Rittman, M., Kuzmeskus, L. B., and Flum, M. A. (1999). A synthesis of current knowledge on minority elder abuse. In Tatara, T. (Ed.), *Understanding elder abuse in minority populations.* Philadelphia, PA: Brunner/Mazel, 221-238.

Smith, J. M. (2000). Race, kinship care, and African American children. Perspectives, Fall 2000, 54-64.

Steinmetz, S.K. (1988). *Duty bound: Elder abuse and family care.* Newbury Park, CA: Sage.

Tatara, T. (1999). Introduction. In Tatara, T. (Ed.), *Understanding elder abuse in minority populations.* Philadelphia, PA: Brunner/Mazul, 1-9.

U. S. Department of Health and Human Services (2000). Report to the congress on kinship foster care. Washington, DC: U. S. Children's Bureau , Contract No #hhs-100-96-0011 (*http://aspe.hhs.gov/hsp/kinr2c00/full.pdf*)

Wolf, R. S. (1988). Elder abuse: Ten years later. *Journal of the American Geriatrics Society*, 758-62.

Yoshihama, M. (2002). *Breaking the web of abuse and silence: Voices of battered women in Japan. Social Work, 47,* 4, 2002, 389-400.

The Elder Abuse
of Custodial Grandparents:
A Hidden Phenomenon

Jordan I. Kosberg, PhD
Gordon MacNeil, PhD

SUMMARY. The abuse of older custodial grandparents is believed to be among the most invisible social problems in society. Using a family systems perspective, the possible abuse of these grandparents is discussed to exist as a result of high risk grandchildren, the vulnerability of older grandparents, and the existence adult children. Custodial grandparents are unlikely to report their abuse by grandchildren; thus, there are profound implications for those from the helping professions. *[Article copies available for a fee from The Haworth Document Delivery Service: 1-800-HAWORTH. E-mail address: <docdelivery@haworthpress.com> Website: <http://www.HaworthPress.com> © 2003 by The Haworth Press, Inc. All rights reserved.]*

KEYWORDS. Custodial careparents, grandchildren, grandparent abuse, family system, vulnerability

---

Jordan I. Kosberg is University of Alabama Endowed Chair of Social Work, School of Social Work, University of Alabama, Box 870314, Tuscaloosa, AL 35487. Gordon MacNeil is Associate Professor, School of Social Work, University of Alabama, Tuscaloosa, AL.

[Haworth co-indexing entry note]: "The Elder Abuse of Custodial Grandparents: A Hidden Phenomenon." Kosberg, Jordan I., and Gordon MacNeil. Co-published simultaneously in *Journal of Elder Abuse & Neglect* (The Haworth Maltreatment & Trauma Press, an imprint of The Haworth Press, Inc.) Vol. 15, No. 3/4, 2003, pp. 33-53; and: *Elder Abuse: Selected Papers from the Prague World Congress on Family Violence* (ed: Elizabeth Podnieks, Jordan I. Kosberg, and Ariela Lowenstein) The Haworth Maltreatment & Trauma Press, an imprint of The Haworth Press, Inc., 2003, pp. 33-53. Single or multiple copies of this article are available for a fee from The Haworth Document Delivery Service [1-800-HAWORTH, 9:00 a.m. - 5:00 p.m. (EST). E-mail address: docdelivery@haworthpress.com].

33

It is an interesting paradox that one of the very first publications focusing upon the problem of elder abuse was entitled "Granny Bashing" (Baker, 1975); yet, almost 25 years later (and a plethora of articles and books on the topic), there has been little written on the abuse of grandparents, especially those raising their grandchildren. While, in the U.S., custodial grandparents raising grandchildren is seen as a somewhat recent phenomenon, it is believed that such childrearing roles for grandparents have been more common in many countries of the world, and brought about by high rates of out-migration by children's parents from rural to urban areas or to other countries to seek greater economic opportunities.

The vulnerability of custodial grandparents to elder abuse (perpetrated by their children and grandchildren) is believed to be a growing phenomenon in the U.S. for many reasons, to be discussed. This article is an antecedent effort to describe the growth of custodial grandparents caring for grandchildren in the U.S., individual and family characteristics that can result in abusive behavior, and the continuing invisibility of abused grandparents.

While the focus of this article is on the U.S., it is believed that the problem of abuse against custodial grandparents is hardly limited to this country and that those from other countries of the world concerned about either custodial grandparenting or elder abuse should "sharpen their focus" to include the potential or existing problem of abused custodial grandparents by their own children and/or their own grandchildren. This article, then, emanates out of the belief that the invisible problem of elder abuse of custodial grandparents is under-studied and not addressed in the literature, and that there is a need for empirical investigation of this most invisible problem.

THE GROWTH OF CUSTODIAL GRANDPARENTS

Grandparents raising grandchildren as result of crises in the family has existed for centuries. They have taken over when their grandchildren were orphaned by disease or war or when financial troubles split a family. They have also stepped in to support single mothers and widowed or divorced parents (Minkler & Roe, 1992). What does appear to be new is a much higher prevalence rate for grandparents raising grandchildren than was seen in the past (de Toledo & Brown, 1995). Although the potential age of these grandparents can range from the mid-30s to 90s, this article focuses upon those who are considered elderly and/or vulnerable.

Who Are They? According to 2000 U.S. Census data, 4.8 million children under age 18 live in grandparent-headed households, an increase of 30% compared to 1990 Census data. This figure represents 6.3% of all children in the U.S. (Tucker, 2002). In a third of these households, neither parent is present (Burnette, 1999). Additionally, Burnette indicates that there is a disproportionate representation of African Americans, Hispanics, low income persons, and those living in urban areas. Grandparents who assume the role of primary caretaker can experience negative consequences, with reported increases in distress, depression, and deteriorating health after the addition of children to the household. Often, the grandparents who assume the caregiving role may also be vulnerable to additional risks of poverty and live in stressful environments (Sclaia, 2002). In order to best understand these consequences, a closer look at the demographic profile of custodial grandparents is necessary.

While households are often comprised of only grandparents and grandchildren, many families in which the grandparent provides custodial care can include three generations. This is to suggest that some households include the child's parent, although the grandparent has custodial responsibilities. The parent may be a minor, have financial problems, and/or has a serious illness or suffered a debilitating accident. It is also possible that there is no difficulty, but the family members choose to live together.

Of families with three generations, a grandparent heads 75% of them (Bryson & Casper, 1999). Half of the grandparent-maintained households have both grandfather and grandmother living with the grandchild. Grandmothers head most of the others. In grandparent-maintained households, 15% of the grandmothers and 21% of the grandfathers are over the age of 65 (Bryson & Casper). While the stereotypical "sandwich" family of the parent maintaining the household while caring for both their children and parents is in evidence, Bryson and Casper found this occurrence to be overstated. They found that the grandparent is likely to be neither elderly, in poor health, nor unemployed. In fact, many of these grandparents are playing an active role in contributing to the family's income and caring for the grandchildren while the parent works. About half of custodial grandparents are still in the workforce (U.S. Census, 2000).

Traditional gender norms in the U.S. often "dictate" that females assume caregiving roles in the family and not remarry when widowed. As a result of their having worked at home or in lower paying positions outside the home, older females are more likely to be non-affluent (compared with their male counterparts). Such issues have led the greater likelihood that single grandmothers will be the caregivers for their grandchildren. So, too, inequities in society result in the fact that these women will head less-affluent households than would grandfathers. Indeed, 60% of grandparent-headed households are grandmother-headed (U.S. Census, 2000), and these households are about twice as likely to be impoverished as are households headed by grandfathers (30% versus 12%). Those families with a male presence (primarily referring to grandfathers) experience much lower rates of poverty. This "pattern" of female-headed, impoverished families with custodial grandparents is most common in African-American families (Bryson & Casper, 1999).

Precipitating Factors. There are a number of factors precipitating custodial grandparenting. Legal mandates that have altered child welfare policies have been associated with increased caregiving by grandparents. In particular, stricter criteria for acts of child abuse, regulations that encourage reporting of suspected child abuse, as well as increased financial reimbursement for familial foster caregiving by grandparents have all resulted in increased rates of caregiving by grandparents (Berrick & Needell, 2000; Minkler & Roe, 1996).

There are numerous social issues that have contributed to this phenomenon. Increasing rates of divorce and teen pregnancy, as well as the effect of drugs (such as crack cocaine) have all had a disrupting effect on nuclear family structures and increasing alternative family structures (Minkler & Roe, 1993; Pruchno, 1999). The inability of parents to raise their children; as a result of their physical and mental health problems, accidents, domestic violence, or death; also contribute to increasing rates of grandparent-maintained households where grandparents are primary caregivers to their grandchildren (Fuller-Thomson, Driver, & Minkler, 1997; Minkler, 1999). Further, the incarceration of parents has lead to more grandparents rearing their grandchildren. In 1991 over 60% of the women incarcerated in federal prisons had minor children, and increasing rates of incarceration for minority females are likely to result in higher rates in following years (Greenfield & Minor-Harper, 1991).

Two additional precipitating reasons for grandparents raising grandchildren deserve special note. First, financial strain sometimes results in a parent relinquishing custody for a child, or children, to a parent. This may or may not be done formally, and may or may not be considered a permanent resolution. In some cases only one or two of several siblings are separated from their parents. While such children may experience the benefits of more personal care, and even more affluence, they may develop feelings of desertion and worthlessness. These feelings may manifest in problem behaviors in the grandparent's household. The second reason for grandparents raising grandchildren relates to teen pregnancy. In this instance, the grandparent is essentially raising two children of very different ages. The teen-parents are likely to be wrestling with issues of their own emancipation while concurrently dealing with issues of responsibility and care for a newborn or infant child. The imposition of authority by the grandparent, who heads the household, may provoke tension, resentment, and even violent behavior by the teen-parent.

Duration of Caregiving Responsibility. The above are various explanations for grandparents being placed in the position of caregiving for their grandchild. Another way of conceptualizing these reasons is to consider that some are short-term situations that require grandparental intervention, such as accidents or work-related circumstances. These precipitating events often occur without warning and require immediate responses and adjustments on the part of the grandparent as well as the grandchild. The incarceration or death of the parent has similar dynamics, although the caregiving is likely to be for an extended period of time. Alternatively, part-time (daycare) supervision by a grandparent may evolve into full-time parenting. This latter scenario is likely to provide a more gradual and less-stressful transition for both the grandparent and the grandchild. A different issue is created by the dynamic of "on-again, off-again" custodial grandparent caregiving. In these situations, the parent fluctuates between being in the grandchild's life and being absent from the child. These fluctuations often occur without warning and of varying lengths of time, and are therefore stressful for the grandparent and grandchild alike.

Aside from the situations that create the need for grandparents to provide custodial care for their grandchildren, most of these care providers do so for personal reasons. Many grandparents report that they are unprepared to accept a child into their house, but do so because they are concerned that the child will be lost to the family if they do not provide custodial care. There can be many phrases that can be heard from grandparents who take on custodial care of a grandchild: "I'm all he has," "We want to keep the kids together," "It don't matter what people say as long as I love you" (Poindexter, 2002). Grandparents are also likely to voice concerns that children placed in institutional care will be "cared for, but not cared about." Thus, it is a sense of responsibility and a need to provide loving care that drives most grandparents to assume the role of primary care provider for their grandchildren.

Least this article perpetuates the myth that all grandparents "live" for their grandchildren, it should be noted that Neugarten and Weinstein (1964) studied 70 grandparents and found five different types of grandparents. Two of the types (distant and traditional) could not be characterized as family-oriented, save in a most minimum manner. While Roberto (1990) believed that the characterization by Neugarten and Weinstein was too "unidemensional," she did acknowledge that all grandparents are not family-oriented. For such persons, the care of grandchildren will not be desired.

Thus, for many different reasons, millions of grandparents are currently raising their grandchildren. While such care has always existed to some extent, the increase in such responsibilities is noteworthy and seems unrelated to socioeconomic status, urban/rural location, or age of grandparents. The tumultuous impact upon older grandparents can be prolific and adversely affect the physical, emotional, social, and economic conditions of older persons. So, too, it is argued, might there be elder abuse.

THE ABUSE OF OLDER PERSONS

Abuse and maltreatment is a problem potentially faced by elderly persons from every socioeconomic status, race and ethnicity, and geographic location (Kosberg, 1988). The problem is world-wide, and exists in developing as well as developed nations. Grandchildren have been found to be less likely to provide care to older relatives that do adult children, and siblings (George, 1986). Yet, the possibility exists and may be growing. Inasmuch as elder abuse has been found to be mainly perpetrated by family members (Administration on Aging, 1998), there is a need to focus upon the children, but also grandchildren of older persons.

Acts of Abuse. Generally, elder abuse is conceptualized to include acts of active and passive neglect, physical and psychological acts, economic and material theft and misappropriation, and denial of rights. Aside from acts of self-abuse, which will not be discussed in this article, research findings have consistently concluded that the major perpetrators of elder abuse are adult children and spouses (Administration on Aging, 1998). The literature concerning grandchildren who abuse their grandparents is quite sparse, although they are included in general discussions regarding "conspiracies" among different members of the family who act together in abusive acts against older relatives.

In 1998, based upon validated reports of elder abuse and neglect from Adult Protective Services (APS) agencies throughout the United States, the Administration on Aging (1998) issued its Final Report on the National Incidence Study. The report indicated that the major category of perpetrators were in the youngest age category (40 and under). Embedded in the statistics, without explanation or discussion, were findings that grandchildren accounted for 9 percent of all elder abuse perpetrators. As broken down by type of abuse, grandchildren accounted for 8.8% of all perpetrators of neglect, 8.9% of all perpetrators of emotional or psychological abuse, 5.6% of all perpetrators of physical abuse, and 9.2% of all perpetrators of financial abuse. As surprising as these statistics might seem, it is believed that these figures are under-estimates of the true incidence of elder abuse by grandchildren.

The Hidden Problem. Kosberg (1988) has suggested that elder abuse is among the most invisible social problems in society. First of all, the problem exists within the home and community representatives may not see the abused person. Indeed, the impaired condition of older persons may preclude their leaving the home. The problem is often seen as a "family affair" and not shared with non-family members. Also, the abused seldom report their adversities to others. For those who are unaware of the problem of elder abuse, there is insensitivity to the existence of the problem and a failure to identity it when it exists.

Research findings have confirmed that grandparents do not readily or easily relinquish their caregiving role for grandchildren (Poindexter, 2002). It might be added that this tenacity seems to prevail regardless of the extent of difficulties brought on by the older person's health problems, economic difficulties, emotional and physical exhaustion, or–it is hypothesized–abuse by the grandchild. Perhaps a bit different than for other types of older abused individuals, custodial grandparents' failure to report adversities (including elder abuse) occurs for several specific reasons, in addition to the general explanations given above. The abused grandparents might be embarrassed that their adult children cannot care for their own children. They might feel guilty that they can no longer provide care for the grandchildren. They might be apprehensive about what will happen to the grandchildren if they are relieved of caregiving responsibilities. Finally, these grandparents might be deterred from relinquishing the caregiving role for grandchildren by their own cultural norms and religious imperatives. The isolation of the grandparent-grandchild dyad, discussed in the literature, also makes the quality of the relationship less visible (Pruchno, 1999). Should abuse occur to the older grandparent, it might be that the abused person will be unwilling to notify others inasmuch as there is a fear of retaliation by the grandchild or belief that there is nothing to be done. Finally, there can be a fear by abused elderly persons that the solution to the problem may be worse than the abuse that they suffer. That is, there may be a fear of being deemed physically or emotionally incompetent, removed from one's home, and institutionalized in a long-long term care facility.

Thus, there is an increased likelihood that grandparents are raising their grandchildren. Given that abuse of these caregivers is difficult to detect, it is concluded that the problem may be much more prevalent that is believed. The following sections will support such a contention, through discussions about the characteristics of many grandchildren that make them high risk for abuse of their caregivers, the characteristics of older custodial grandparents which make them vulnerable to abusive behavior, and appearance by the parents of the children in the caregiving setting. First, however, this article will discuss research findings and social science theory regarding the family and intergenerational family relationships.

FAMILY SYSTEMS PERSPECTIVES

There is a rich body of theory that aids in the understanding of the dynamics involved in the potential abuse of custodial grandparents by their grandchildren and by their adult children who have parented the grandchildren. Goodman and Silverstein (2001) allude to the fact that the absence of strong emotional bonds between family members can result in serious conflict. While affection, shared values, and positive contact all contribute to intergenerational solidarity, such positive values do not always exist within families. Thus, in the first instance, it is necessary to focus upon the quality and commonalities of intergenerational relationships.

Cycles of family violence have been discussed whereby children are raised in violent families and grow up to perpetuate their learned intra-family (and extra-family) interactions (Bandura, 1977). Such families can be considered as dysfunctional, and it has long been known that dysfunctional families produce abused children who are high risk to abuse others (i.e., spouse, their own children). Brogden and Nijhar (2000), writing about elder abuse, state: "Either dysfunctional families characterized by inter-generational violence ensure the cyclical reproduction of elder abuse–parents batter children who in turn abuse the parents in their old age, or elder abuse is spouse abuse grown old" (p. 77). The children learn violence in their formative years in the home and repeat it later as part of a "cycle of violence." It is reasonable to extend such reasoning to grandparents, as well as parents.

Another explanation for such intergenerational transmission of family violence involves learned behavior whereby young children observe the conflict between parents, or their parent and another adult, and the parent and the child are "educated" about the way to interact with others in particular situations. "Many observers have concluded that domestic violence such as child abuse and neglect and spouse abuse is learned in the home and passed from one generation to the next . . ." (Quinn & Tomita, 1997, p. 107). These authors refer to an early study by Straus, Gelles, and Steinmetz (1980) that determined that men who had witnessed a parent abuse another were three times as likely to hit wives as others. This was almost as true for wives. It seems reasonable to assume that children who witnessed the abuse of a parent (whether by the parent's spouse or significant other) are also more likely to abuse a grandparent caring for them.

Cultures of violence are said to exist in particular racial or ethnic groups. There may be empirical support for higher rates of violence focusing upon members of the family as well as outsiders. While cultural explanations might have some relevance, often it is the socioeconomic status and not the racial or ethnic background of family members within a cultural group that seems more important in differentiation rates of family violence. Indeed, often the racial or ethnic background of individuals is misinterpreted by the "cause" of differences in behavior when, upon closer investigation, it is socioeconomic background and not the color of one's skin or country of origin (Weinick, Zuvekas, & Cohen, 2000; Connell & Gibson, 1997).

Attachment theory has also provided some insight into a family systems model to explain the abuse of older family members by those who are younger. Simply put, the quality of interaction between a young infant and the attachment figure (usually the mother) has prodigious implications on the behavior and personality of the developing infant (see Cassidy & Shaver, 1999). Ainsworth (1972) has described three types of attachment: Secure, anxious-ambivalent, and anxious-avoidant. Through childhood and adolescence, continuing through young adulthood and beyond, the type of attachment influences the individual's interaction with classmates, dating behavior, marriage, mental stability, and relationship with family members. Attachment theory has been applied to the relationship between an elderly parent and an adult child caregiver (Cicirelli, 1991), but needs to be empirically tested as an explanation for elder abuse.

HIGH RISK GRANDCHILDREN

Grandchildren raised by grandparents vary greatly in age from very young infants through adolescents to young adults and older adults. In many instances there may be more than one grandchild being cared for by a grandmother (or much less-frequently a grandfather) (Burton, 1992). It is possible that a custodial grandparent will be caring for the grandchildren from more than one child. There is a plethora of research findings and practice experience on the adverse consequences on grandparents who raise their grandchildren that include attention to physical and mental health, stamina and endurance, financial resources, and loss of autonomy and independence to pursue interests, among others (Minkler & Roe, 1996; Burton, 1992).

In particular, the literature has focused upon the health problems of grandchildren that can add to the caregiving demands for grandparents. For example, Minkler and Roe (1996) and Roe and Minkler (1998-1999) have written extensively about grandparents who were "surrogate parents for grandchildren with special needs; prenatally exposed to alcohol or drugs or who were physically or emotionally abused by their parents prior to coming into the grandparent's care" (p. 35). Additionally, they wrote that grandchildren often suffered from hyperactivity, respiratory problems, and other physical and emotional symptoms that could result in difficulties to the grandparents. These writers failed to identify the additional possibility of intentional grandparent abuse by these "special-need" grandchildren. Indeed, only indirectly have such discussions dealt with the possibility that grandchildren might either intentionally or unintentionally abuse their caregiving grandparents. It is believed that there are ample reasons to be concerned about such possibilities.

Creighton (1991) has pointed out that grandchildren who had been "emotionally" or physically abandoned by their parents (and are then cared for by grandparents) "are among the most needy, most emotionally damaged and most angry in the nation" (p. 80). It is a reasonable conclusion that this anger can be directed to the custodial grandparent who serves as an authority figure. Certainly, caring for an adolescent grandchild with emotional problems can place an older, and possibly vulnerable, grandparent at some peril for elder abuse.

In discussing custodial grandparenting of difficult children, Silver-thorn and Durrant (2000) describe grandchildren's oppositional defiant disorder (ODD) and conduct disorder (CD) and give attention to the need for psychological treatment and therapeutic services for grandchildren. They do not, however, address the vulnerability and the needs of caregiving grandparents of such children. Similarly, Baker (2000) focuses upon grandchildren diagnosed with attention-deficit/hyperactivity disorder (ADHD) that results in "low frustration tolerance, temper outbursts, bossiness, stubbornness, demands for immediate gratification, mood lability, demoralization, dysphoria, rejection by peers, and poor self-esteem" (p. 149). However, Baker does not address the potential for violence of custodial grandparents at the hands of the grandchildren. These characteristics of grandchildren are potentially dangerous and related to abusive acts against the others, whether a teacher, a counselor, or a grandparent!

There is a possibility that a grandparent will care for a grandchild who has serious physical, mental, developmental, or cognitive problems, such as retardation, chronically mentally ill, or severe learning disorders (McCallion & Janicki, 2000). While the needs of such children will exacerbate caregiving responsibilities leading to greater caregiving burdens, the possibility of unintentional abusive behavior directed to the grandparent needs to be considered. In an article on "psychological distress" of grandparents (Kelley & Whitley, 2003), the point is made that grandparents are at "significant risk for psychological distress, often serious enough to warrant psychiatric intervention" (pp. 136-137). The special needs and problems of grandchildren will heighten the caregiving burdens, and it is believed that such "significant risks" include the possibility of abuse and maltreatment as well.

Also, with increased frailty of the grandparents comes increased vulnerability for abuse by their specially-challenged grandchildren. Indeed, with medical advances, there is a greater chance that an ailing grandparent might become increasingly dependent upon a grandchild. As such, a type of role reversal may occur. This may pose a very serious threat to the older grandparent, for there is no assurance that a grandchild with have the necessary skills, motivation, or time to provide effective and humane care, or whether elder abuse, neglect, or maltreatment will result.

In her research study comparing two racial groups of caregiving grandparents, Pruchno (1999) found that grandchildren in both groups had a range of behavior problems: Changes in mood or feeling, being nervous or high strung, being argumentative, having trouble paying attention, being hyperactive, being stubborn, demanding attention, demonstrating a disobedient manner at home. Black children were found to be more argumentive, impulsive, felt worthless, unhappy, withdrawn, dependent, and acted too young for their age. "Black respondents were more likely than white respondents to indicate that their grandchild lied or cheated, was disobedient at school, destroyed his or her things, and got into fights" (p. 215).

Yet, Pruchno indicated that the similarities between the two groups of grandmothers were "striking," in terms of background, reasons for caregiving, lack of support, impact upon employment, and positive levels of satisfaction. In fact, it was found that black grandmothers were more likely to have more friends to call upon, received more formal services, and felt less trapped in their role, tired, isolated and alone than did the white grandmothers. Once again, though, there is a need to determine whether or not it is the race and ethnicity of grandparents and/or socioeconomic status.

Adolescent grandchildren may be likely to engage in financial abuse against a grandparent. The desire, if not demand, for spending cash may exceed the ability of the grandparent to provide such financial resources. There is a dearth of empirical findings of grandchildren financially victimizing their grandparents. Yet, findings from studies on financial abuse of older persons lead to the conclusion that family members do steal and misappropriate finances and resources from elderly relatives (Sanchez, 1996; Kalter, 1995), Recall that the Administration on Aging (1998) survey had found that 9.2% of all financial abuse was perpetrated by grandchildren. Thus, there is reason to believe that some grandchildren steal from their grandparents and otherwise coerce them into silence about the theft of finances. One mechanism of coercion (recently told to a co-author by a social worker) involves the grandchild threatening to report being sexually abused if the grandparent did not turn over money to the grandchild, when demanded.

VULNERABILITY OF CUSTODIAL GRANDPARENTS

Most adults do not anticipate becoming custodial grandparents, and this unexpected development will subject them to numerous problems that they would not otherwise encounter. Grandparents who acquire the parental role again are subjected to individual and family life realties that likely differ from what they have expected for their later years. Rather than looking forward to retirement and a lessening of familial responsibility, custodial grandparents are required to devote more energy to these responsibilities. Associated with this atypical, and to some extent unexpected, life trend are physical, psychological, social, and financial strains.

Persons beyond the age of 40 are generally thought to be more susceptible to physical degeneration and illness than are younger persons who are charged with the demanding tasks of parenting. It is therefore no surprise that becoming the parent again is physically challenging for grandparents. The physical endurance required keeping up with toddlers, youth, and adolescents may lead to physical problems for grandparents. Custodial grandparents commonly report increased psychological stress when they become the primary authority figure to youngsters (Burton, 1992; Dowdell, 1995). Accepting increased familial responsibilities, especially the day-to-day care of children, may result in isolation and fewer opportunities for socializing with same-age peers for many custodial grandparents (Minkler, Roe, & Price, 1992).

There is little question that raising grandchildren imposes financial strains on grandparents. The amount of money that government agencies may provide to offset the cost of family foster care is notoriously insufficient to meet the real costs of providing adequate care for these youths. As noted above, females (who are the primary care providers of minors) are more likely to be impoverished than are males. All too frequently, grandparents expend their entire life savings in order to meet the financial demands of providing for their minor grandchildren. Even after they have successfully launched their grandchildren into adulthood, these grandparents suffer the long-range financial consequences of this relationship.

The stresses and problems experienced by grandparents who become the primary caregivers of their grandchildren are also experienced as lifestyle changes (Dowdell, 1995). Their relationships with other adult children may be altered. Also, extended family members may be affected by new roles. For instance, children living with one set of grandparents may experience reduced encounters with the other set of grandparents. Other lifestyle changes in work, social life, and recreational activities may result from the presence of grandchildren in the home (Dowdell, 1995). Certainly the dreams and aspirations of grandparents are impacted by their assuming primary caregiving responsibilities. Along with the financial, legal, health, and psychological factors resulting from this new role, the grandparent and grandchild are also typically forced to wrestle with emotions concerning the precipitating event that led to this new family structure, whether it is death, incarceration or rejection of the parent.

Acknowledged is the high-risk nature of many grandchildren cared for by their grandparents and the lack of attention given to the possibility of grandparent abuse. There is an extensive literature on the abuse of children, spouses, and older persons; yet, the professional attention given to older abuse victims has generally failed to address the possibility of elder abuse of vulnerable grandparents by their grandchildren. As one example, an issue of the American Society on Aging journal, *Generations* (1998-1999) was devoted to intergenerational dynamics within the family. The primary article in that issue related to abusive family relationships, entitled "Older Persons at Risk," by Hirshorn and Piering, failed to discuss the possibility of abuse of grandparents by their grandchildren.

High-risk profiles exist that identify older persons who can be considered especially vulnerable for abuse and maltreatment (Kosberg, 1988). Such general profiles can identify high-risk custodial grandparents. The great majority of grandparents who raise grandchildren are females who may be less able to defend themselves from abuse (Bryson & Casper, 1999). The literature on custodial grandparents has consistently found low levels of strength, stamina, and endurance that, in turn, make them vulnerable to acts of commission against them (Kosberg, 1988). Additionally, emotional or physical exhaustion may make the older grandparent more dependent on the grandchild. Female caregivers are more susceptible to adverse consequences of caregiving, such as depression and anxiety (Miller & Cafasso, 1992). Phillips et al. (2000) have written about the vulnerability of older caregiving women to the abuse by those for whom they give care. These authors identify such abusers as spouses or parents, and do not address the possibility of abuse of caregiving grandmothers at the hands of their grandchildren.

A body of research focuses upon the "burden" experienced by grandparents raising their "high risk" grandchildren. In these studies vulnerability focuses upon physical and/or emotional consequences resulting from the caregiving responsibilities. For example, Dowdell (1995) assessed the consequences of raising grandchildren with regard to family support, physical and mental health problems, personal time and scheduling, and the perception of emotional stress. Burton (1992) focused upon such consequences as depression or anxiety, increased smoking and drinking, heightened medical problems, slight stroke, and multiple stressful outcomes. In both studies, there was no attention to the consequences of abuse and maltreatment by the grandchildren.

The vulnerability of some grandparents may be exacerbated by culture. Phillips et al. (2000) compare older Hispanic (generally Mexican) and non-Hispanic caregivers. Within the former culture there is believed to exist a higher rate of intra-family aggression, as explained by use of strict discipline of children, masculine superiority, emphasis on submission and obedience to authority figures, separation of sex roles, father dominance, and strong gender-role differentiation. If at all accurate, the role of such cultural values begs for an answer to the implications of male dominance, gender role differentiation, and strong discipline of children within a family context where grandchildren are raised by older (primarily female) grandparents.

Burton (1992) studied black grandparents raising children of drug-addicted parents and described three levels of stressors facing these grandparents. The first level, *Contextual*, pertains to the existence of crime and violence within grandparent's neighborhood. The second level, *Familial*, deals with the multidimensional drains upon the grandparent as a result of caring for several family members. The third level of stressor, *Individual*, focuses upon the unique consequences to grandparents, such as challenges to freedom, independence, and self-determination. The possibility of adverse behavior by grandchildren is not mentioned. The reader is reminded that Pruchno (1999) had found significant similarities between black and white grandmothers and that it may be that blacks have more formal and informal support systems upon which to use. It is also necessary to consider whether it is racial background or socioeconomic status that might be related to differences between different groups of caregivers.

Toledo et al. (2000) also addressed the normative values faced by different family members of Hispanic families that can include a combination of respect for elders (respeto), male ideal (macho), selflessness of the women (abnegation), and trust between members of the family (confianza). Such a conceptualization for "harmonious" relationships between different generations of male and female members of a family may not always exist, and may be challenged by differences in levels of adherence to cultural norms between different generations in the family as a result of the acculturation of the younger members of the family.

Somewhat relatedly, Clarke et al. (1999) have written about conflicts (differences) between older parents and adult children. The areas of conflict include; (1) communication and interaction styles, (2) habits and lifestyle choices, (3) child-rearing practices and values, (4) religion, politics, and ideology, (5) work habits and orientation, and (6) household standards or maintenance. If these differences between the two

generations of elderly parents and their adult children can result in conflicts, what intergenerational conflicts might there be between older
grandparents and their young grandchildren?

Admittedly, custodial grandparents are, in the main, grandmothers.
Yet, there is a need to consider the gender of both grandparents and
grandchildren. Creasey and Koblewski (1991) studied adolescent
grandchildren's relationships with grandparents and concluded that
granddaughters held more positive relationships with their grandparents, and that grandmothers received more positive regard than grandfathers. Male members of the family may be caregivers (Kramer &
Thompson, 2002) and it may be assumed–given increased breakdown
of gender-specific normative roles in society–that grandfathers may become more prevalent in raising grandchildren in the future. Boxer,
Cook, and Cohler (1986) found that peer group values, socioeconomic
status, and acculturation have significant influence in determining relationships between three generations of male relatives, including male
grandchildren and grandfathers. They caution against measuring men
by "a feminine ideal." As will be discussed, there is little known about
the quality of relationships between grandfathers caring for grandchildren, either with or without a spouse.

Creasey and Koblewski (1991) and Hodgson (1992) studied the importance of gender of grandchildren and grandparents and came to a
similar finding that grandmothers receive more positive regard than do
grandfathers. Goodman and Silverstein (2001) included parents of
grandchildren in a study of close relationships between grandmothers
and grandchildren. Among other findings was the conclusion that
where there were harmonious relationships between "triads" (of three
generations) there was less stress for grandmothers. The Goodman and
Silverstein article focused upon female triads and the question of the
consequences when there might be males among any one of the triad
members remains to be determined.

ADULT CHILDREN OF CUSTODIAL GRANDPARENTS

The parents (fathers or mothers) of grandchildren under the care of
grandparents may add additional complexity to the possibility of abuse.
It may be that the parent (or parents) of the children dwell in the community within which live the caregiving grandparent(s) and care recipient grandchildren. These parents may periodically visit their children
(and caregiving parents). This is to suggest that children's parents may

not have caregiving responsibilities due to an inability to perform childrearing tasks (i.e., substance abuser, mentally ill) or being unavailable to undertake such responsibilities (i.e., incarceration, hospitalization), but they may none-the-less contribute a powerful influence in the family dynamic.

The existence of the children's parents might be an additional source of abuse against the custodial grandparents. These adult children might seek to engage in abusive behavior out of their guilt in not caring for their own children, embarrassment at having to rely on their aging parents to care for their children, or anger directed to the aging parents for a variety of reasons. The grandparents may not wish their adult children to visit their grandchildren, inasmuch as the grandchildren may become overly disruptive, angry, or depressed after seeing their parents. Indeed, there may be legal restrictions to the parent interacting with the grandchild at all, regardless of the grandparent's preference on the issue.

Additionally, adult children, especially those who have social and/or psychological pathologies or economic problems, have been found to be high risk to abuse older parents (Kosberg, 1988). Any intergenerational conflict between the parent of the grandchild and the grandparent is likely to reinforce conflicts between grandchild and grandparent. Should the adult child be dependent upon the older parents, the possibility of anger, and abuse, is increased. Thus, adult children in addition to grandchildren should be seen to be potential abusers of custodial grandparents.

APPLIED IMPLICATIONS

Mills (2001) suggests that work on assessing dynamics within the family, including the relationships between grandparents and grandchildren, suffers by a narrow perspective by researchers and clinicians. "Methodological limitations include the use of small and non-inclusive samples, most of which pertain to only one or two generations. Yet, there are now more three-, four-, and five-generation families, and multiple family forms. As a result, the grandparent role has become more complex, with the possibility of multiple grandparent roles such as great-grandparents and great-great-grandparents" (p. 679).

The implication is that while there is increased attention to the role of custodial grandparents and the challenges they can face, the dynamics might become evermore complex. There are prodigious responsibilities for professionals to assist these caregivers (Roberto & Qualls, 2003).

This chapter cannot address the preventive and interventive efforts that should be created to assist, encourage, and support custodial grandparents. Some books with such a purpose have been published (de Toledo & Brown, 1995; Kornhaber, 1996). A welcome addition to the literature in this area is a recent text edited by Hayslip and Patrick (2003) that focuses upon specific programmatic efforts for grandparents. Hooyman and Kiyak (2002) have illustrated the issues facing custodial grandparents: Legal, financial, childcare, medical insurance, schooling, and psychological challenges to both the grandchild and the grandparent. What is yet to appear is literature on the methods by which to prevent abuse of custodial grandparents and by which to intervene when they are abused.

While there is a great need for increased professional attention to the needs of custodial grandparents, in general, there is an additional need to become sensitive, aware, and concerned about the possibility of the abuse of these grandparents. This article is an antecedent effort to call attention to the possible existence of such problems, problems that have not been addressed by those who focus upon the problem of elder abuse and maltreatment.

Research is needed to determine if and how custodial grandparent abuse is different from other forms of elder abuse with regard to antecedents and consequences. From findings should follow necessary efforts to support, assist, and–in come cases–replace custodial grandparents who not only face emotional demands, health related consequences, but also abusive acts against them. But, inasmuch as the problem exists, there is a need for immediate awareness by those in the helping professions and those who advocate on behalf of older persons.

REFERENCES

Administration on Aging (2003). *The national elder abuse incidence study: Final report (September 1998).* http://www.aoa.gov/abuse/report/default.htm

Ainsworth, M.D.S. (1972). Attachment and dependency: A comparison. In J.L. Gewirtz (Ed.), *Attachment and Dependency.* (pp. 97-137). Washington, DC: Winston.

Baker, A.A. (1975). Granny battering. *Modern Geriatrics 8*: 20-24.

Baker, D. B. (2000). Custodial grandparenting and ADHD (pp. 145-160). B. Hayslip Jr., & R. Goldberg-Glen (Eds.), *Grandparents Raising Grandchildren: Theoretical, Empirical, and Clinical Perspectives.* New York: Springer Publication Company.

Bandura, A. (1997). *Social Learning Theory.* Englewood Cliffs, NJ: Prentice-Hall.

Beerick, J. D., & Needell, B. (2000). Recent trends in kinship care: Public policy, payments and outcomes for children. In P.A. Curtis, & D. Grady, (Eds.), *The Foster*

Care Crisis: Translating research into policy and practice. Washington DC: Child Welfare League of America and University of Nebraska Press.

Boxer, A.M., Cook, J.A., & Cohler, B.J. (1986). Grandfathers, fathers, and sons: Intergenerational relations among men (pp. 93-121). In Pillemer, K.A., & Wolf, R.S. (Eds.), *Elder Abuse: Conflict in the Family.* Dover, MA: Auburn House Publishing Company.

Brogden, M., & Nijhar, P. (2000). *Crime, Abuse, and the Elderly.* Portland, OR: Willan Publishing.

Bryson, K., & Casper, L.M. (1999). *Coresident Grandparents and Grandchildren:* U.S. Bureau of the Census, Population Division Working Paper No. 26/ Washington, DC: U.S. Bureau of the Census.

Burnette, C. (1999). Physical and emotional well-being of custodial grandparents in Latino families. *American Journal of Orthopsychiatry 69*: 305-318.

Burton, L.M. (1992). Black grandparents rearing children of drug-addicted parents: Stressors, outcomes, and social service needs. *The Gerontologist 32*(6): 744-751.

Cassidy, J., & P.R. Shaver (1999). *Handbook of Attachment: Theory, Research, and Clinical Applications.* New York: The Guilford Press.

Cicirelli, V.G. (1991). Attachment theory in old age: Protection of the attached figure (25-42). In K. Pillemer, & K. McCartner, (Eds.), *Parent-Child Relations Throughout Life.* Hillsdale, NJ: Lawrence Erlbaum Associates.

Clarke, E.J., Preston, M., Raksin, J., & Bengtston, V.L. (1999). Types of conflicts and tensions between older parents and adult children. *The Gerontologist 39*(3): 261-270.

Connell, C.M., & Gibson, G.D. (1997). Racial, ethnic, and cultural differences in dementia caregiving: Review and analysis. *The Gerontologist 18*(2): 92-100.

Creasey, G.L., & P.J. Koblewski (1991). Adolescent grandchildren's relationships with maternal and paternal grandmothers and grandfathers. *Journal of Adolescence 14*: 373-387.

Creighton, L.L. (1991). Silent saviors. *U.S. News and World Report 111*(25).

DeToledo S., and Brown, D.E. (1995). *Grandparents as Parents: A Survival Guide for Raising a Second Family.* New York: The Guilford Press.

Dowdell, E.B. (1995). Caregiver burden: Grandmothers raising their high-risk grandchildren. *Journal of Psychosocial Nursing & Mental Health Services 33*(3): 27-30.

Fullmer-Thompson, E., Driver, D., & Minkler, M. (1997). A profile of grandparents raising grandchildren in the United States. *The Gerontologist 37*: 406-411.

George, L.K. (1986). Caregiver burden: Conflict between norms of reciprocity and solidarity. In K.A. Pillemer, & R.S. Wolf, (Eds.), *Elder Abuse: Conflict in the Family.* Dover, MA: Auburn House Publishing Company.

Goodman, C.C., & Silverstein, J. (2001). Grandmothers who parent their grandchildren. *Journal of Family Issues 22*(5): 557-578.

Greenfield, L. A., & Minor-Harper, S. (1991). *Women in prison.* Washington, DC: Bureau of Justice Statistics.

Hayslip, B. Jr., P. Silverthorn, R. J. Shore, & C.E. Henderson (2000). Determinants of custodial grandparents' perceptions of problem behavior in their grandchildren (255-268). B. Hayslip Jr., & R. Goldberg-Glen (Eds.), *Grandparents Raising Grand-*

children: Theoretical, Empirical, and Clinical Perspectives. New York: Springer Publication Company.

Hirshorn, B., & Piering, P. (1998-1999). Older people at risk: Issues and intergenerational responses. *Generations XXII*(4): 49-53.

Hodgson, L.G. (1992). Adult grandchildren and their grandparents: The enduring bond. *International Journal of Aging & Human Development 34*(3): 209-225.

Hooyman, N.R., & Kiyak, H.A. (2002). *Social Gerontology: A Multidisciplinary Perspective* (6th ed.). Boston: Allyn and Bacon.

Kalter, J.M. (1995). I trusted him. *New Choices for Retirement Living 35*(1): 66.

Kelley, S.J., & Whitley, D.M. (2002). Psychological distress and physical health problems in grandparents raising grandchildren: Development of an empirically based intervention model. In B. Hayslip Jr., & J.H. Patrick, (Eds.), *Working with Custodial Grandparents*. New York: Springer Publications.

Kornhaber, A. (1996). *Contemporary Grandparenting*. Thousand Oaks, CA: Sage Publications.

Kosberg, J.I. (1988). Preventing elder abuse: Identification of high risk factors prior to placement decisions. *The Gerontologist 28*(1): 43-50.

McCallion, P., & Janicki, J. (2000). *Grandparents as Carers of Children with Disabilities: Facing the Challenges*. New York: The Haworth Press, Inc.

Miller, B., & Cafasso, L. (1992). Gender differences in caregiving: Fact or artifact? *The Gerontologist 32*(4): 498-507.

Mills, T.L. (2001). Grandparents and grandchildren: Shared lives, well-being, and institutional forces influencing intergenerational relationships: An epilogue to the special issues. *Journal of Family Issues 22*(5): 677-679.

Minkler, M., Roe, K.M., & Price, M. (1992). The physical and emotional health of grandmothers raising grandchildren in the crack cocaine epidemic. *The Gerontologist 32*(6): 752-761.

Minkler, M., & Roe, K.M. (1996). Grandparents as surrogate parents. *Generations XX*(1): 34-38.

Neugarten, B.L., & Weinstein, K. (1964). The changing American grandparent. *Journal of Marriage & the Family 26*(2): 199-204.

Phillips, L.R., Torres de Ardon, E., & Solis Briones, G. (2000). Abuse of female caregivers by care recipients: Another form of elder abuse. *Journal of Elder Abuse & Neglect 12*(3/4): 123-143.

Pillemer, K.A., & Wolf, R.S. (1986). *Elder Abuse: Conflict in the Family*. Dover, MA: Auburn House Publishing Company.

Poindexter, C.C. (2002). "It don't matter what people say as long as I love you": Experiencing stigma when raising an HIV-infected grandchild. *Journal of Mental Health & Aging 8*(4): 331-348.

Pruchno, R. (1999). Raising grandchildren: The experiences of Black and White grandmothers. *The Gerontologist 39*(2): 209-221.

Quinn, M.J., & Tomita, S. K. (1997). Elder Abuse and Neglect: Causes, Diagnosis, and Intervention Strategies (2nd ed.). New York: Springer Publishing Company.

Roberto, K.A. (1990). Grandparent and grandchild relationships. In T.H. Brubaker, (Ed.), *Family Relationships in Later Life*. Newbury Park, CA: Sage Publications.

Roberto, K.A., & Qualls, S.H. (2003). Intervention strategies for grandparents raising grandchildren: Lessons learned from thee caregiving literature (13-26). In B. Hayslip, Jr., & J.H. Patrick (Eds.), *Working with Custodial Grandparents.* New York: Springer Publishing Company.

Roe, K.M., & Minkler, M. (1998-1999). Grandparents raising grandchildren: Challenges and Responses. *Generations XXII* (4): 25-32.

Sanchez, Y.M. (1996). Distinguishing cultural expectations in assessment of financial exploitation. *Journal of Elder Abuse & Neglect 8*(2): 49-59.

Scalia, R. (2002). Helping "kinship care"-givers. *Social Work Today,* December 9, 2002:15.

Silverthorn, P., & Durrant, S.L. (2000). Custodial grandparenting of the difficult child: Learning from the parenting literature (47-63). In B. Hayslip Jr., & R. Goldberg-Glen, (Eds.), *Grandparents Raising Grandchildren: Theoretical, Empirical, and Clinical Perspectives.* New York: Springer Publication Company.

Straus, M.A., Gelles, R., & Steinmetz, S.K. (1980). *Behind Closed Doors: Violence in the American Family.* Garden City: NY: Anchor/Doubleday.

Toledo, J.R., Hayslip Jr., B., Emick, M.A., Toledo, C., & Henderson, C.E. (2000). Cross-cultural differences in custodial grandparenting (107-144). In B. Hayslip Jr., & R. Goldberg-Glen, (Eds.), *Grandparents Raising Grandchildren: Theoretical, Empirical, and Clinical Perspectives.* New York: Springer Publication Company.

Tucker, C. (2002). Grandparents raising grandchildren: The child care solution? *Social Work Today,* December 9, 2002: 12, 14-15.

Weinick, R.M., Zuvekas, S.H., & Cohen, J.W. (2000). Racial and ethnic differences in access to and use of health care services, 1977 to 1996. *Medical Care Research and Review 57*(Sup. 1): 36-54.

Combating Elder Financial Abuse–
A Multi-Disciplinary Approach
to a Growing Problem

Betty Malks, MSW, CSW
Jamie Buckmaster, BA
Laura Cunningham, MPA

SUMMARY While the number of violent crimes in the United States is decreasing, financial crimes against the elderly are increasing due to the aging of the overall population and greater concentration of wealth among older people. The United States, along with the rest of the world, is experiencing dramatic growth of its senior populace; and financial abuse of the elderly is also dramatically rising. Santa Clara County, California's response to this problem via their model program emphasizing a

---

Betty Malks is Director, Department of Aging and Adult Services, Santa Clara County Social Services Agency, 591 North King Road, San Jose, CA 95133 (E-mail: Betty.Malks@ssa.co.santa-clara.ca.us). Jamie Buckmaster is Social Services Program Manager, Adult Protective Services, Santa Clara County Social Services Agency, 591 North King Road, San Jose, CA 95133 (E-mail: Jamie.Buckmaster@ssa.co.santa-clara.ca.us). Laura Cunningham is Senior Management Analyst, Department of Aging and Adult Services, Santa Clara County Social Services Agency, 591 North King Road, San Jose, CA 95133 (E-mail: Laura.Cunningham@ssa.co.santa-clara.ca.us).

The authors would like to acknowledge the valuable assistance of James Ramoni and Michelle Woldridge.

[Haworth co-indexing entry note]: "Combating Elder Financial Abuse–A Multi-Disciplinary Approach to a Growing Problem." Malks, Betty, Jamie Buckmaster, and Laura Cunningham. Co-published simultaneously in *Journal of Elder Abuse & Neglect* (The Haworth Maltreatment & Trauma Press, an imprint of The Haworth Press, Inc.) Vol. 15, No. 3/4, 2003, pp. 55-70; and: *Elder Abuse: Selected Papers from the Prague World Congress on Family Violence* (ed: Elizabeth Podnieks, Jordan I. Kosberg, and Ariela Lowenstein) The Haworth Maltreatment & Trauma Press, an imprint of The Haworth Press, Inc., 2003, pp. 55-70. Single or multiple copies of this article are available for a fee from The Haworth Document Delivery Service [1-800-HAWORTH, 9:00 a.m. - 5:00 p.m. (EST). E-mail address: docdelivery@haworthpress.com].

multi-disciplinary approach to combating financial abuse will be discussed. *[Article copies available for a fee from The Haworth Document Delivery Service: 1-800-HAWORTH. E-mail address: <docdelivery@haworthpress.com> Website: <http://www.HaworthPress.com> © 2003 by The Haworth Press, Inc. All rights reserved.]*

KEYWORDS. Financial Abuse Specialist Team (FAST) Model Program

The purpose of this paper is to provide the professional community with an overview of Santa Clara County's Financial Abuse Specialist Team (FAST) protocol for this model program. FAST is a unique and innovative multi-disciplinary collaboration designed to combat elder financial abuse. The emphasis is on rapid response and the ability to intervene and freeze assets before the elder or dependent adult becomes financially destitute. The Financial Abuse Specialist Team was developed to address the growing problem of financial abuse within Santa Clara County and has been effective in meeting the needs of the community.

The U.S. Department of Justice, Office of Victims of Crime has recognized the Department of Aging and Adult Services' FAST Team, and has offered to be the focal point for the distribution and marketing of the video nationwide. This collaboration will provide local governments with a blueprint for replicating FAST rapid response as a model program in their own communities. The FAST video can be obtained by anyone, free of charge, by calling the Department of Justice's Office of Victims of Crime 1-800-627-6872 or visiting the Department of Justice, Office of Victims of Crime Website *<http://puborder.ncjrs.org>*. The videotape number is NCJ198153.

As of February 2004, FAST has prevented the loss of and/or recovered $106.1 million, which includes: Prevention of loss of $65,512,800 million in real property, $24,874,054 million in liquid assets, $7,185,569 million in stocks and bonds; and $8,529,319 in restitution orders.

INTRODUCTION

The United States along with the rest of the world is experiencing dramatic growth of its senior population. While the number of violent crimes in the U.S. is decreasing, financial crimes against the elderly are increasing due to the aging of the population and greater concentration of wealth among older people. According to Wasik (2002), elder financial abuse is quickly becoming the crime of the 21st century as demonstrated by research of his own as well as statistics from the National Center on Elder Abuse (1998): It is estimated only 1 in 14 incidences of abuse is reported, and with financial abuse it is estimated to be 1 in 100; Elders are likely to hide abuse because of shame, humiliation and fear of retaliation, or placement in a nursing home; 60-90% of the perpetrators of financial abuse are family members or in-home care givers; Since persons over 50 control at least 70% of the nation's (U.S.) household net worth, they are frequent targets for exploiters; Victims are typically female, frail and mentally impaired. Seventy-five percent are between the ages of 70 and 89.

Recommendations for Addressing Abuse

In response to this growing problem, the first national conference to address issues of elder abuse in ethnic minorities was initiated and organized by Action on Elder Abuse, United Kingdom and the Neighborhood Care Project (Newham) Ltd., United Kingdom. During the course of this conference, recommendations were made to resolve this issue. Many of the recommendations are already incorporated in the Financial Abuse Specialist Team practices. Those recommendations made by the council and which are the fundamental components of FAST practices are as follows: (1) There is a need for information and training about elder abuse for older people, their families, and caregivers and for ethnic minority groups. (2) There is a need for partnership building and joint working among social work, housing and health authorities. (3) There is a need to establish multidisciplinary working groups on elder abuse (*SPEAKING OUT: National conference on elder abuse within minority communities, 1998*).

Santa Clara County's Response–Best Practices Model Overview

Launched in May 1999 in response to the growing problem of financial abuse among the elder and dependent adult population within Santa Clara County, FAST has become a model program for combating financial abuse. FAST is a multi-disciplinary collaboration comprised of four teams with representatives from the Department of Aging and Adult Services' (DAAS) Adult Protective Services (APS) and Public Administrator/Guardian/Conservator (PAGC); the District Attorney's office

(DA), and the County Counsel. Interdisciplinary teamwork has been the key ingredient in achieving FAST goals. The fundamental components of FAST are: (1) FAST responds within hours, and is available 24 hours a day, seven days a week. (2) The rapid response component is critical to the early intervention of financial abuse. Early intervention often facilitates favorable case resolution and avoids costly and protracted criminal and civil litigation. (3) Through FAST action, in addition to preserving financial assets, steps are taken to improve living arrangements and create greater independence, broader choices regarding medical care, and enhanced physical and emotional health.

FAST's innovation centers around three key elements: (1) The multi-agency team–a partnership that increases each member's effectiveness. (2) Rapid response and the ability to freeze assets–facilitates favorable case resolution and avoids costly and protracted litigation. (3) The collaborative will and ability to address all aspects of clients' well being.

FAST has been in existence for four years and has developed a law enforcement protocol and is in the process of developing a protocol for financial institutions. The protocols will address a multitude of financial abuse scenarios which will enable the team to move forward and effectively address issues.

FAST is committed to the prevention of financial abuse regardless of the size of the estate. FAST has always taken the position that a person's Social Security check and/or pension check is as important to him/her as a larger amount is to a person who has an estate worth millions. Cases are prioritized by the imminent danger of loss and/or risk and the presence of a looming predator, not the overall amount of the estate.

The Vulnerability Quotient

Santa Clara County has a high incidence of financial abuse, is an affluent community, and has a large elderly population. This combination of circumstances has resulted in the development of the vulnerability quotient. As the elderly population increases, so will the incidence of financial abuse, particularly in a state with skyrocketing real estate. California is a state of great prosperity and is considered the 5th largest economy in the world. Santa Clara County has one of the highest median incomes among metropolitan areas in the nation.

According to the Bay Area Census (2002), the median income for a family of four is $84,663. According to the San Jose Mercury News, the median price of a single family home in November of 2003 was approximately $520,000. In high property value areas such as this one, housing prices have made senior homeowners highly vulnerable to exploitation even when they have little disposable income and few other financial assets. Statistics in Santa Clara County for 2002 reflect of all adult abuse reports made, financial abuse constituted 32% of the total reports (657) as represented by the attached graph.

Because of the many factors addressed above, Santa Clara County has a high vulnerability quotient (see Graph 1). Two factors that strongly influence the vulnerability of financial abuse victims are:

Increased Aging Population + Concentration of Wealth Among Older People = Financial Abuse Vulnerability.

This high vulnerability quotient led Santa Clara County to develop the Financial Abuse Specialist Team (FAST), a unique multi-disciplinary model which emphasizes prevention as the key to addressing this problem. As you will see, this model incorporates many of the elements recommended by the National Conference on Elder Abuse including education, partnership and multi-disciplinary teams.

The FAST Protocol

According to Malks, Schmidt, and Austin (2002), new legislation (State of California Senate Bill 2199 enacted in 1999) and the increasing incidence of financial abuse were the driving forces in the development of the FAST team protocol. The following is a history of the development of the team, case flow, as well as a review of the emergency response and litigation component:

GRAPH 1. Santa Clara County Financial Abuse Reports–2002

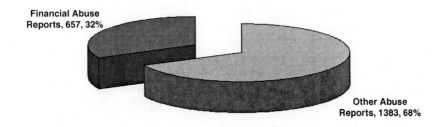

Financial Abuse
Reports, 657, 32%

Other Abuse
Reports, 1383, 68%

History

Two occurrences drove the development of FAST: California's legislation, Senate Bill 2199, that standardized APS programs statewide. One of the requirements of this legislation was APS' immediate response to life threatening situations and/or situations of imminent danger. The rise in financial abuse cases accounting for 30% of all reported cases in Santa Clara County at that time and the philosophy that rapid response is the key to recovery and prevention created the urgency to develop a new practice model.

The Department of Aging and Adult Services took a proactive approach to the implementation of this new legislation by convening the APS stakeholders committee. Forty-six community advocates came together to make recommendations regarding the redesign of APS in Santa Clara County to better fit community needs.

A toll free 24-hour abuse reporting number was established. An outreach campaign was developed utilizing all media formats giving examples of elder abuse and neglect and encouraging people to call the toll-free number to report suspected fraud or abuse. Systems were put in place to provide tangible support services for victims. The policy to implement 24/7 response was based on the Senate Bill 2199.

The passage of this legislation also created new State funding for Adult Protective Services and multi-disciplinary teams. These multi-disciplinary teams, such as FAST, continue to be sustained by both state and county funds. FAST currently uses existing staff from each discipline who volunteer for assignment on the team.

Based on the new legislation and the ensuing increase of financial abuse to 30% of all abuse cases, FAST Rapid Response was implemented in May 1999 to provide immediate response for investigating and acting on reports of financial abuse in Santa Clara County. According to the California Welfare and Institutions Code, FAST is considered a multi-disciplinary personnel team, meaning "any team of two or more persons who are trained in the prevention, identification, and treatment of abuse of elderly or dependent persons and who are qualified to provide a broad range of services related to abuse of elderly or dependent persons" (Welfare and Institutions Code, Section 15753.5, 1999).

In addition to the rapid response and crisis intervention components, the establishment of FAST provided the community with both a deterrent to prevent future incidents of financial abuse and the ability to move quickly to prevent losses by creating a seamless service delivery system.

DAAS selected members for the FAST team (APS social workers, PAGC investigative staff, DA staff and County Counsel) by asking for volunteers. Team members were selected based on their skills in problem-solving and crisis intervention. Due to the nature of their work, APS social work staff was less familiar with the financial aspects involved. County Counsel provided training to APS Social Work staff on such matters as trusts and estates. Training continues on an on-going basis as necessary.

Case Flow

Graph 2 shows the typical flow of a financial abuse case from the beginning of the process to case resolution. Calls are often generated from relatives or friends of the alleged victim as well as from police, neighbors, attorneys, community-based organizations, and/or caregivers. Reports may originate from a number of different sources, and the reporting party's identity is always confidential. Reports may also originate in the Public Administrator/Guardian's office or the DA's office. All calls are then transferred to APS. Other reports may be a result of a direct call to APS. Once a call comes in, it is screened by an APS social worker to obtain basic information, determine if financial abuse seems likely, and if there is imminent danger. The referral is then reviewed by an APS supervisor who decides how to proceed. After-hours emergency calls are handled by an on-call social worker. If the case is assessed as not being urgent, it is sent to a bi-weekly review committee consisting of staff from each of the four agencies. Staff reviews the case for evidence of abuse. If evidence is found or it is decided further investigation is needed, the case is referred to the FAST team.

Emergency Response

If the APS supervisor reviews the report and determines there may be a need to act quickly due to potential loss of property, a referral form is faxed to the PAGC intake worker who then logs the referral and forwards it immediately to the PAGC Inquiry Screener. A joint visit is made to interview the alleged victim and make an assessment. The practice is for at least two team members to go out at all times. These team members will make a joint determination (based on the allegations in the original referral) as to whether the DA Investigator should be included at this time. Once the team has interviewed the alleged victim, they conduct a mini-mental status exam (MMSE) of the victim. This is a

GRAPH 2

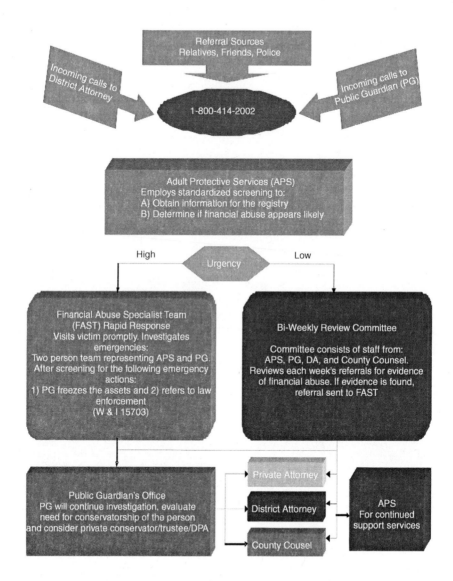

screening tool that gives team members a first glimpse into the victim's mental status. If the alleged victim appears to be cognitively impaired or subject to undue influence, the team may choose to take the following actions:

1. File a certificate under California Probate Code 2901. This provision allows the alleged victim's assets to be frozen by the Public Administrator/Guardian's office.
2. File for emergency temporary conservatorship. In Santa Clara County, this can happen the same day.
3. Ask a physician to file a Medical Declaration form that attests to the alleged victim's incapacity, and/or refer to law enforcement.

California Probate Code 2901 states that when filing a certificate to freeze assets the following guidelines apply:

1. A Public Administrator/Guardian staff member who is authorized to take control of the property under this chapter may issue a written certification of that fact. This certification is effective for fifteen days after the date of issuance.
2. The Public Administrator/Guardian is authorized to record a copy of the written certification in any county where real property is located or which the Public Administrator/Guardian is authorized to take possession or control under this chapter.
3. A financial institution or other person shall, without the necessity of inquiring into the truth of the written certification and without court order or letters being issued:

   1. Provide the Public Administrator/Guardian information regarding property held in the sole name of the proposed ward or conservatee.
   2. Surrender to the Public Administrator/Guardian property of the proposed ward or conservatee that is subject to loss or misappropriation.

4. Receipt of the written certification:

   1. Constitutes sufficient acquaintance for providing information and for surrendering property of the proposed ward or conservatee.

2. Fully discharges the financial institution or other person from any liability as a result of any act or omission of the Public Administrator/Guardian with respect to the property.

Once temporary conservatorship is established, the Public Administrator/Guardian's office is obligated to investigate and determine if there is a need for appointing a permanent conservator. Private conservators are considered and although another party may eventually be appointed as conservator, the team remains involved providing continued services and assisting in any legal proceedings that may commence.

Legal Component

Under the Welfare and Institutions code, Adult Protective Services is required to report any suspected criminal activity to law enforcement, and law enforcement is required to cross-report abuse and/or neglect to APS.

When it is determined that sufficient documentation and evidence exist of illegal activity or undue influence on the part of the suspected abuser, the legal professionals of the multi-disciplinary team pursue the case. The legal members of FAST are the District Attorney who will prosecute the crime, and the County Counsel who may continue the conservatorship process for the Public Guardian's office and may bring forth any civil litigation on behalf of a conservatee. Investigation into the suspected criminal act can occur by law enforcement or the district attorney's investigators, who are also law enforcement officers. Each is assigned to gather information and interview people to assist in obtaining a conviction of the suspected abuser.

As mentioned earlier, the DA Investigators for FAST usually go out into the field with another member of the team. This allows for separate interviews of the victim and the suspected abuser, which can be critical to investigating the alleged crime. The team can also identify any immediate needs of the client, as well as, gather further information regarding client assets and financial documents. If assets have not been frozen by the Public Guardian under California Probate Code 2901, the priority of the team at this time is to ameliorate the financial abuse as quickly as possible, using other strategies such as case work intervention, law enforcement support and collaboration with financial institutions in order to ensure the well-being of the client. Recent legislation has allowed law enforcement to videotape victims for use in court, if necessary. This has been enormously helpful to the prosecution of crimes if the older adult later becomes confused, demented or passes away.

Collateral contacts may be made with the assessor's office regarding any real property owned by the client and any recent transactions that have occurred. Depending on the situation, further interviews may be needed with relevant collateral contacts including family, neighbors and friends of the victim and/or suspect. Search warrants may be issued for bank records. The evidence is then presented to the deputy district attorney assigned to FAST who has the necessary expertise to prosecute financial abuse cases.

He/she reviews the case and decides what charges are appropriate. A complaint is completed, sent to the criminal court and is reviewed by a judge who subsequently signs the warrant and sets bail. At that time, or a later time, the judge may sign an order requiring that information be provided regarding the source of the bail money. In addition, the judge may issue a restraining order requiring the suspected abuser to stay away from the victim. The law enforcement agency that investigated the case then receives the arrest warrant. Once the suspected abuser is detained, there are several legal steps that will occur. It is up to the district attorney's office to not only prosecute the case but consider restitution and recovery for the victim. As previously detailed in this document, prevention of financial abuse is key; however, the proactive prosecution, restitution and recovery aspects of the FAST model are critically important (Malks, Schmidt, and Austin, 2002).

It should be noted that one of the dilemmas in prosecuting financial abuse cases is the desire of the victim to protect the alleged abuser who may be a relative or more likely, his/her own adult children. This may occur because of the victim's denial, reliance by the elder on that same abuser for care and support, fear of retaliation, or placement in a nursing home. In addition, the elder may have lost the ability to deal with their own finances and may not fully understand what has occurred.

Because of the rapid response component, this best practices model can do more to prevent and/or recover losses. FAST pursues these crimes, prosecutes these criminals, and has successfully returned property and assets to elders in the amount of $106.1 million.

However, there are other types of financial abuse that FAST encounters which are equally as financially debilitating to the elder. FAST also deals with scams as an additional threat to the financial security of our elderly population. Typically, scams prey on the frail elderly who are alone and isolated and may include a perpetrator professing romantic interest and using undue influence to separate the elder from family and friends (sweetheart scam) or using fraudulent telemarketing or e-mail techniques (Canadian Lottery and Nigerian scams) to convince elders to give them money.

FAST Case Histories

The following are actual cases taken from FAST files:

Mr. H.

The 86-year-old Mr. H., whose name has been changed to protect his identity, came to live with his daughter in Santa Clara County after his wife died in Hawaii. Before long, his daughter amended his trust to name herself as co-trustee, prevailed upon him to deed a $300,000 beachfront cottage in Hawaii to her, had two vehicles transferred to her name, and made out checks totaling $85,000 to herself and her family members.

Meanwhile, the County Adult Protective Services began an investigation in response to allegations that his daughter was verbally and financially abusing him, and was about to kidnap and flee with him against his will to Hawaii. Mr. H. lacked capacity and FAST obtained temporary conservatorship of Mr. H. and transferred his bank accounts and trust out of the daughter's name into his own.

Mrs. G.

Mrs. G. is a wealthy 89-year-old widow whose husband passed away the previous year after 65 years of marriage. Mrs. G. and her husband had been affluent members of the community and, later after he retired, they became great philanthropists. In the years prior to his death, Mr. G. had befriended a younger man at a local coffee shop. The younger man quickly became a friend to the couple. No longer able to do many of his same activities around their large home, Mr. G. turned them over to the younger man. Eventually the younger man began isolating the couple from friends and relatives. After the husband's death, the suspected abuser moved into the home and began to ingratiate himself further into the widow's life. He eventually took over her financial affairs and began to liquidate her accounts.

Adult Protective Services received a report of suspected abuse regarding the suspected abuser's attempts to liquidate the assets. FAST responded immediately. The team discovered Mrs. G. was cognitively impaired by administering the Mini-Mental Status Exam (MMSE), one of the tools used for assessment. Her doctor was contacted and concurred with FAST that Mrs. G. had moderate dementia. The doctor completed a medical declaration.

It was agreed that FAST would move forward with conservatorship in order to protect her assets. The assets were frozen using CA Probate Code 2901, and a temporary conservatorship was issued. The suspected abuser became belligerent and threatened County staff and law enforcement. An EPRO (emergency protective order) was issued by law enforcement, 24-hour care was put in place for Mrs. G., and a bodyguard was hired to protect her. Later, a permanent conservatorship was granted.

PROGRAM ENHANCEMENTS

Financial Institutions Project (FIT)

The addition of financial institutions to FAST's repertoire of strategies to combat elder financial crime has been the most recent augmentation to the program. Recently, Santa Clara County's Department of Aging and Adult Services and local financial institutions announced the launching of a campaign to increase awareness of financial abuse of seniors. The goal of the campaign is to increase knowledge about the escalating threat of financial abuse among our elderly population and to enhance prevention efforts. This collaborative effort is referred to as the Financial Institutions Training Project (FIT). Its objective is to encourage financial institutions to work closely with the Financial Abuse Specialist Team (FAST) in formulating and initiating a plan to train financial institution staff in recognizing possible at-risk persons or situations, and to reinforce the importance of early detection.

In the past, credit unions and banking institutions had been challenged by what to do in situations of potential elder or dependent adult financial abuse. One of the first credit unions to recognize this problem was Star One, located in Sunnyvale, California. Managers and employees noticed that handling at-risk members would require special training and careful approach. As a result, Star One Credit Union established the Beneficiary and Retiree Services (BRS) group to address the emerging issues. Through education and practice, the BRS group formed a model that is still followed by Star One today. With this model for early detection of financial abuse, employees are more equipped and better prepared to face the challenges of sensitive member service situations and their legal ramifications, such as privacy concerns.

Due to their reporting of several cases to Santa Clara County Adult Protective Services, Star One was viewed as the starting place to forge an alliance between the financial industry and the local social service agencies. The interdependency and exchange of information proved so crucial in getting help to the members of Star One, that the APS and BRS group started meeting face to face. Over time, this relationship grew into a stepping stone for launching the bigger project. Today, other credit unions and banks in the County have joined the partnership of APS and Star One to form the Financial Institutions Project Team. They include Golden Bay FCU, Mission City FCU, Meiwest, Peninsula Postal CU, Santa Clara FCU, Technology CU, Valley CU, and Wells Fargo Bank. The participation of many financial institutions will be a key component in locating individuals that prey on the elderly and strip them of their financial assets.

Law Enforcement Protocol

The Department of Aging and Adult Services brought together the 15 local law enforcement agencies, plus the coroner, victim witness program, the long-term care ombudsman program, and the District Attorney's office to create and implement a most comprehensive law enforce- ment protocol for the investigation of abuse and neglect perpetrated towards elders and dependent adults. This is a step by step guide to assist law enforcement in responding to elder and dependent adult abuse calls. The office of the California Attorney General has announced that they will use the Santa Clara County law enforcement protocol as an example for the state.

RESULTS

FAST has assisted victims in sustaining their quality of life and independence. FAST has been the recipient of several local and national awards as well as a grant from the Federal Department of Justice, Office of Victims of Crime, to produce a video that would provide agencies nationwide with an instructional tool for replicating Santa Clara County's

Financial Abuse Specialist Team (FAST) protocol. The production and dissemination of the FAST video has allowed the team to share its expertise in the development and implementation of a unique and innovative multi-disciplinary collaboration.

CONCLUSION

Several factors including the passage of California Senate Bill 2199, an increase in the number of financial abuse reports, and the high vulnerability quotient led Santa Clara County to develop FAST, a unique multi-disciplinary model which emphasizes prevention as the key to addressing elder financial abuse. The establishment of FAST provided the community with both a deterrent to prevent future incidents of financial abuse and the ability to move quickly to prevent losses by creating a seamless service delivery system. Since attitudes among elders vary and are based on cultural perspective, more research is needed so that we may better understand the impact of cultural differences on the prevalence and incidence of abuse. FAST's future includes: (1) Enhancing the Law Enforcement protocol and continued training of law enforcement officers (2) Developing a financial institutions protocol and training financial institution employees. (3) Training the faith based community.

Preliminary plans for a formal evaluation include the creation of an evaluation policy group and the services of a professional evaluator who would guide the process. The chief goals will be to determine how we can measure both the qualitative as well as quantitative benefits of FAST. The process would begin by a distribution of surveys to practitioners and management staff to obtain feedback about what is working and what is not working. Also, there is a need to evaluate the consistency of the team's responsiveness and assess equitability of partners/team utilization to determine if there is effective use of resources. Also, more research is needed on FAST's efficacy and methods of operation. Currently a policies and procedures handbook is in the process of being developed. The evaluation process will allow us the opportunity to review and improve our methods of operation in order to refine service delivery and ensure client well-being.

REFERENCES

Bay Area Census. (2002). Retrieved from *http://census.abag.ca.gov/counties/Santa ClaraCounty02.htm*

California Probate Code 2901. Retrieved from *http://www.leginfo.ca.gov*

California Welfare and Institutions Code. (1999). Section 15753.5. Retrieved from *http://www.leginfo.ca.gov*

Malks, B., Schmidt, C., Austin, C. (2002). Elder Abuse Prevention: A Case Study of the Santa Clara County Financial Abuse Specialist Team (FAST) Program. *Journal of Gerontological Social Work*, Vol. 39 (3), 30-35.

McAllister, S. (2003). Santa Clara County home sales up 39%. *The Mercury News*. Retrieved from *http://www.bayarea.com/mld/mercurynews/2003/11/21/business/7316745.htm*

National Center on Elder Abuse. (1998). *The National Elder Abuse Incidence Study*. Retrieved from *http://www.elderabusecenter.org/default.cfm?p=nis.cfm*

SPEAKING OUT: National conference on elder abuse within ethnic minority communities. (1998). Convened by Action on Elder Abuse, UK, Neighbourhood Care Project (Newham) Ltd. UK. Retrieved from *http://www/aeweb.org/conference%20 reports/London. htm*

Wasik, J.F. (2000). The Fleecing of America's Elderly. *Consumer Digest*. March/April, 78-79.

Study of Elder Abuse
Within Diverse Cultures

Jordan I. Kosberg, PhD
Ariela Lowenstein, PhD
Juanita L. Garcia, EdD
Simon Biggs, PhD

SUMMARY. The article provides an overview of the challenges to cross-cultural and cross-national research on elder abuse. There are conceptual and methodological difficulties in undertaking comparative studies within and between countries. As an example of the need to address cultural diversity within a country, elder abuse efforts in the U.S., UK, and Israel are described. The most pressing need for cross-national research on abuse involves a common definition of such adversities

---

Jordan I. Kosberg is University of Alabama Endowed Chair of Social Work, School of Social Work, University of Alabama, Box 870314, Tuscaloosa, AL 35487. Ariela Lowenstein is Professor and Director, Center for Research and the Study of Aging, Faculty of Social Welfare and Health Studies, Haifa University, Haifa, Israel. Juanita L. Garcia is Adjunct Professor, College of Human Environmental Sciences, University of Alabama, Tuscaloosa, AL. Simon Biggs, is Professor, Centre for Social Gerontology, School of Social Relations, Keele University, Keele, UK.

This study is an adaptation of "Challenges to the Cross-Cultural and Cross-National Study of Elder Abuse" that appeared in the *Journal of Social Work Research and Evaluation 3*(1), 2002 (pp. 67-31); Springer Publishing Company, Inc., NY 10012. Used by permission.

[Haworth co-indexing entry note]: "Study of Elder Abuse Within Diverse Cultures." Kosberg, Jordan I., et al. Co-published simultaneously in *Journal of Elder Abuse & Neglect* (The Haworth Maltreatment & Trauma Press, an imprint of The Haworth Press, Inc.) Vol. 15, No. 3/4, 2003, pp. 71-89; and: *Elder Abuse: Selected Papers from the Prague World Congress on Family Violence* (ed: Elizabeth Podnieks, Jordan I. Kosberg, and Ariela Lowenstein) The Haworth Maltreatment & Trauma Press, an imprint of The Haworth Press, Inc., 2003, pp. 71-89. Single or multiple copies of this article are available for a fee from The Haworth Document Delivery Service [1-800-HAWORTH, 9:00 a.m. - 5:00 p.m. (EST). E-mail address: docdelivery@haworthpress.com].

http://www.haworthpress.com/web/JEAN
10.1300/J084v15n03_05

against the elderly that is reflective of the values within a country and at a sufficient level of discourse to embrace diverse conceptualizations of the problem. *[Article copies available for a fee from The Haworth Document Delivery Service: 1-800-HAWORTH. E-mail address: <docdelivery@haworthpress.com> Website: <http://www.HaworthPress.com> © 2003 by The Haworth Press, Inc. All rights reserved.]*

KEYWORDS. Cross-cultural, cross-national, comparative analyses, elder abuse definitions

Elder abuse is a problem identified in both developing and developed nations (Kosberg & Garcia, 1995). Studies on the problem have used different definitions, methodologies, and populations (Kozak, Elmslie, & Verdon, 1995; Schiamberg & Gans, 1999), making it difficult to merge findings that, in turn, would lead to more definitive conclusions about the causes and consequences of elder abuse. Moreover, as knowledge is cumulative, building research findings upon earlier ones also becomes problematic as these methodological differences multiply within what is often assumed to be a homogeneous research base. Not only is the comparative analysis of elder abuse adversely affected by conceptual and methodological problems, but the sharing of preventive and interventive efforts to combat this problem is also made more tenuous when there are differences in the definition of the problem within and between different countries. This article focuses upon cross-national research on elder abuse and seeks to determine whether there can be conceptual models to be used for the study of elder abuse in different populations within and between countries.

Toward such an end, researchers in the U.S., UK, and Israel began a dialogue focusing upon the possibility of conducting a comparative international study of elder abuse that would address both conceptual and methodological issues. Each of these three countries has heterogeneous populations including a sizeable group of immigrants from differing and contrasting cultures who face a variety of social, economic, and political problems. There are differences in these countries that challenge comparative approaches in the study of elder abuse.

CULTURAL DIVERSITY

The complexities of elder abuse studies result from not only variations in definitions of the phenomena, but are also due to the cultural diversity of populations within a country. Elder abuse studies from such countries as the U.S., Canada, UK, and Israel, in particular, have intentionally or inadvertently included participants from different cultural backgrounds. In some instances, elder abuse studies have failed to identify the implications of the variations in cultural backgrounds of those studied in a particular country. But even when such is done, there is little notice taken of the diversity within a particular cultural group. For example, Hispanic and Asian populations in the U.S., Sephardic Jews in Israel, or those of Indian backgrounds in the UK are more dissimilar than they are alike.

Consider the heterogeneity among such Hispanic populations as rural Mexicans in Texas, upper class Cuban Americans in Miami, and middle class Puerto Ricans in New York City. In Israel, Moroccan Jews who came to Israel 20 years ago share little with Ethiopian Jews who have recently arrived. Consider what is common between British-born Asians and those who have experienced multiple homelands, Silheti Bangladeshis in the most deprived part of East London and Sikhs or Punjabi Hindus in the middle-class suburbs of Bradford. The point could be made that African Americans from the upper class in Atlanta, the middle class in Los Angeles, and the lower class in rural Mississippi share little in common. In Israel, upper class Christian Arabs living in Nazareth are quite unlike the rural Moslem group living in Daburia. However different these cultural groupings may be, they are often–whether insensitively or naively–put together under a common ethnic or racial heading within a large study.

There are also obvious challenges in translating measurement instruments for different populations in any one country in the effort to have identical meanings in the different languages. So, too, there is a need to guard against the inappropriate superimposing of the researcher's values and norms from one cultural background on the studied populations from others. For example, in a study of cultural meanings in the assessment of financial exploitation, Sanchez (1996) concludes that there must be awareness by researcher and practitioner alike of the cultural realities and meanings of certain forms of adversity. She suggests that the researcher's definition of financial exploitation may not correspond with that of subjects' cultural expectations and experiences. Quoting Sanchez (1996): "The failure to recognize the distinctness of exploitation and the nature of interactions within a heterogeneous population has resulted in a limited understanding of this issue, *thus creating the need to consider differing perspectives"* (p. 57, emphasis added).

In the U.S., Annetzberger, Korbin, and Tomita (1996) found that the perception of the existence and severity of elder abuse differed between those representing different cultural backgrounds (i.e., Japanese Americans, Mexican-Americans, Korean Americans, African-Americans). Whether or not differences in perceptions equated with actual differences in the incidence of abuse requires more rigorous empirical study, as differences between groups might have been based upon the meaning and importance of the questions being asked, as well as the actual differences in perceptions.

In studies of the influence of ethnicity or race on individual attitudes or behavior, it is necessary to determine whether it is the racial or ethnic background of a group that is predictive of negative attitudes and behavior toward older persons. Possible alternative explanations may be related to religion, religiosity, social class, geographic location, family characteristics, social class, and degree of acculturation. Connell and Gibson (1997) indicate that making comparisons by racial group is inherently problematic as what is attributed to race might well be social class, or cultural or historical background. Kozak, Elmslie, and Verdon (1995) discuss contradictory findings about the prevalence of elder abuse and neglect in White and African American populations that they attribute to an inability to ensure that the two samples were equated on other factors (e.g., socioeconomic status). Lawton et al. (1982) found that younger, better educated, and more affluent African American caregivers experienced higher levels of burden than older, less educated, and less affluent African Americans, thus suggesting that race alone is insufficient to predict attitudes or behaviors.

As an indication of a growing awareness that the dynamics surrounding elder abuse vary within different subcultures in the U.S., the National Center on Elder Abuse, along with the American Public Welfare Association and the Archstone Foundation, sponsored a national conference on Understanding and Combating Elder Abuse in Minority Populations. The conference included sessions on African Americans, Hispanics, Asian Pacific Islanders, American Indians, as well as other groups.

In a similar fashion, the Center for Research and Study of Aging at Haifa University in Israel, together with a geriatric rehabilitative hospital and a Haifa municipal unit of aging, has organized parallel conferences and workshops comparing various ethnic groups within the Jewish society as well as Jewish and Arab subpopulations. Recently, there was a national conference on elder abuse in Israel that included Arab, along with Jewish, professionals.

In Israel, it would seem important to control for not only religion, but also the type (and extent) of religious affiliation; inasmuch as differences range from liberal reform to ultra-orthodox within the Jewish population. Indeed, any discussion of Israelis must make some distinction between Arabs and Jews, the Jews with European backgrounds and Jews of other origins, Israeli sabras (native-born) and recent immigrants, as well as distinct living arrangements (i.e., urban areas, rural small town, or kibbutz communities).

In the UK, attempts have been made, conceptually, to include cultural and ethnic diversity within the study of elder abuse by a variety of governmental and social policy organizations. There have also been a number of books, from a variety of positions, outlining, summarizing, and re-defining cultural issues of elder abuse (Biggs, Kingston, & Phillipson, 1996; Bennett, Kingston, & Penhale, 1997). Until very recently (Penhale 2003), there has been an absence of a political willingness to fund empirical research on abuse. British research has had to rely on a small number of early inquiries into institutional mistreatment and inspection reports on residential and nursing care (Kingston, 2003). As with the Israeli experience, U.S. and Canadian research has been drawn on heavily in the UK with little consideration as to its transferability and appropriateness, or to the heterogeneity of the studied population.

British studies need to recognize the diversity of the experience of migration and the intergenerational similarities and differences of experience that might result, in addition to the complexity of arrangements within and between groupings. In the London Borough of Harringay (a geographical/administrative unit of approximately 500,000 people), for example, it is possible to encounter 26 language groups along with accompanying differences in culture and experience.

There are methodological considerations with regard to the sampling frame of national studies, inasmuch as findings on elder abuse are often extrapolated from a biased sample to a community, state, regional, or national community and, thus, may be criticized for over-generalizing. In a study of the use of long-term care services by frail elders in the U.S. (Mui & Burnette, 1994), race and ethnicity (along with age and sex) were found to be predisposing variables to outcome measures. The authors admit that their non-random sample of volunteers possibly resulted in sample biases. Additional questions can be raised regarding the sampling of groups from particular backgrounds (i.e., whites, middle class, urban). Acknowledging the more privileged populations often studied (in retirement research), Calasanti (1996) suggests that attention given to less powerful strata of society will yield more valid definitions of social reality than from more powerful respondents.

CROSS-NATIONAL STUDIES

Similar to challenges in research across racial and ethnic groups within a country are those faced by researchers undertaking cross-national studies of elder abuse. Guidance can be provided by the work on other comparative topics. Smith (1994) has written about the difficulties in comparative studies of the health and economic status of elderly persons in developing countries with regard to the existence of comparable and reliable data, as well as the use of differing definitions. Smith also alludes to differences between objective current data and subjective retrospective data on measurements of health.

In a book on child maltreatment, Knudson (1992) identifies specific limitations with various data collection techniques. Data from self-reports depend upon recall and truthfulness (and cognitive ability), data from observations of maltreatment may reflect professional biases (or being unaware of the adversity), data from reports based upon professional or layperson observations allow for a broad definition of adversity but depend on a willingness to report and includes only observed acts; and data from investigated reports are dependent upon recorded information, are limited by observations of the phenomenon, influenced by investigator turnovers, and permit only a short-term view. Ogg and Munn-Giddings (1993), writing about research methodologies in studies of elder abuse in Great Britain and the U.S., have also identified similar challenges resulting from different data collection techniques. Cross-national research on elder abuse, or in any such comparative study, requires the existence of reliable and valid data, independent of its source.

Shaw et al. (1997) attempted a cross-cultural validation of coping strategies and caregiver distress in Shanghai, China and San Diego, California. After common instruments were deemed to be reliable, differences were found between the two locales, and the lower levels of Chinese caregiver adversity were explained by cultural differences with regard to family interdependence, veneration of elderly family members, and acceptance of the traditional family role. This study has ramifications for the consideration of international studies of elder abuse, inasmuch as findings indicate that low levels of caregiver coping were related to high levels of caregiver distress (which can be related to elder abuse). Also, there is a need to find comparable measurement instruments in different countries (and determine the reliability of such instruments), and there is the need to validate the translation of instruments from one language (culture) to another language (culture).

As with the study of subpopulations within a country, cross-national studies of elder abuse, too, must consider the characteristics of the participants who are studied and then compared. Calasanti (1996), addressing the diversity of different experiences (such as retirement) by different groups (for example, by race or ethnicity) emphasizes the importance of power (those who have it and those who are oppressed by it). She suggests that international-level comparisons need to incorporate sensitivity to the influence of one's "Westernized" biases in definitions and methodologies, and also to understand the cultural norms and mores in other countries within which comparative studies are being undertaken.

Finally, in reviewing studies of elder abuse reported in Ireland, France, and the Nordic countries, Canadian writers (Kozak, Elmslie, & Berdon, 1995) have stated: " . . . little detailed information is available to permit one to say more than that the phenomenon exists" (p. 138). Thus, cross-national comparative analyses may be limited at this time to descriptive studies rather than to more rigorous explorations based upon conceptual or theoretical frameworks.

VARIATIONS IN THE DEFINITION OF ELDER ABUSE

The need to avoid "Westernized biases" in the definition of elder abuse, and factors related to the problem, poses a challenge to researchers. Even in the U.S., there have been significant differences in the definition of elder abuse (Schiamberg & Gans, 1999). One of the co-authors (Kosberg, 1988) has defined the problem of elder abuse to include passive and active neglect, physical (including sexual) mistreatment, psychological abuse, theft or misappropriation of finances and/or possessions, and denial of rights. Some American studies include maltreatment within institutional settings as a form of abuse (Pillemer & Moore, 1989); others have not (Kosberg & Nahmiash, 1996), and some studies include self-abuse (Bozinovski, 2000), while other studies include only cases where there is at least abusing and abused persons (Pillemer & Finkelhor, 1989). In Britain, attempts to define abuse and neglect have also been subject to contradictory demands and have evidenced a tendency to extend the meaning of abuse until it ceases to have precision

(Brammer & Biggs, 1998). Recent attempts to achieve an internationally valid definition, such as that taken by the World Health Organization, in collaboration with the International Network for the Prevention of Elder Abuse (2002), may go some way to increase agreement on the scope and comparative validity of the phenomenon (Biggs, 2003).

Researchers undertaking comparative analyses of elder abuse in various countries are challenged to consider definitions from other countries along with their own. One book (Kosberg & Garcia, 1995) that presents descriptions of elder abuse in ten different countries (Australia, Finland, Greece, Hong Kong, Israel, India, Ireland, Norway, Poland, and South Africa) found diversity in definitions of elder abuse as well as differences in the level of concern and awareness. So, too, were there similar conclusions by Biggs and Kingston (1995) in a special edition on elder abuse in *Social Work in Europe* (which included articles on Norway, France, Spain, Italy, the Netherlands, Ireland and the UK).

As an example of the variations which exist between countries in the definition of elder abuse, the Kosberg and Garcia book (1995) disclosed that elder abuse in Norway includes "family disharmony" (Johns & Hydle, 1995), in Hong Kong it includes "elder dumping" (Kwan, 1995), and in India includes "disrespect" by a daughter-in-law (Shah, Veedon, & Vasi, 1995). Hugonot (1990) reports that 20% of French elderly experience "moral cruelty" in the home (in Kozak, Elmslie, & Verdon, 1995). Given strong values for Filial Piety in the Far East, and elsewhere, the placement of an elderly relative into an institutional setting–a relatively recent phenomenon–might be considered an example of elder abuse (Chan, 1985). Indeed, not too long ago the high suicide rate among elderly person in Japan was attributed to the introduction of institutional placements used as an alternative to relieve tensions between wives and their mothers-in-law (Kaneko & Yamada, 1990; Soeda & Araki, 1999). On the other hand, given a tradition of public responsibility for the care of elderly persons in Sweden, it has been suggested that turning to family caregiving (seen as economically-advantageous by government) can be perceived to be abusive by both older persons and their families (Johansson, 1997). Such variations in the definition of abusive behavior between countries, as well as within countries, necessitate the consideration of conceptual frameworks for elder abuse that can embrace such diversity. Admittedly, research on elder abuse in different countries of the world has adopted the definitions and explanations for abuse from, in the main, American, Canadian, and British studies. As the study of elder abuse increases around the world, it can be expected that there will be a "protest" against these earlier definitions, and an understandable desire to create definitions congruent with a country's own situation. In Australia, as one example, Dunn and Sadler (1993) and McCallum (1993) have argued for a unique conceptualization of the causes of elder abuse that better reflects the "Australian character." Indeed, the path to awareness of the existence of elder abuse, and then on to research studies of the problem, varies by country.

ELDER ABUSE IN THREE COUNTRIES: U.S., ISRAEL, AND U.K.

The international study of elder abuse in the world has not changed greatly over the years from early descriptive studies using definitions and methodologies developed in the U.S. Yet, the motivation to undertake comparative analyses of elder abuse in two or more countries is believed laudable. It is important to determine the unique and common features in elder abuse within different countries, so to move closer to a determination of whether or not there are universal factors–as opposed to culturally-influenced factors–that either directly lead to, or indirectly contribute to, the problem of elder abuse.

The U.S. The emergence of work on elder abuse in the U.S. began the late 1970s and early 1980s (Kosberg, 1988) and accelerated in the latter 1980s and 1990s. While elder abuse was initially defined to include only adversities occurring in private dwellings in the community perpetrated by a member or members of the elderly person's informal support system (family, friends, or neighbors), abuse within congregate and institutional settings was included at the end of the 1980s (Pillemer, 1988). Work on elder abuse varied over the years from surveys that extrapolated from Adult Protective Service data (Tatara, 1993), studies that involved the identification of high risk indicators of elder abuse (Pillemer, 1986; Kosberg & Nahmiash, 1996), or those that utilized case records or expert judgments on the existence of elder abuse (Lau & Kosberg, 1979; Rosenblatt, 1996). Theoretical explanations for elder abuse most often included a list of theories or models (i.e., social exchange, symbolic interaction, environmental press) extrapolated to elder abuse. With the exception of a presentation comparing elder abuse in Hong Kong and the U.S. (Kosberg & Kwan, 1989), which consisted of a description of elder abuse in both countries, there were few efforts at cross-national comparisons of elder abuse.

Israel. The study of elder abuse in Israel began in the late 1980s (Lowenstein, 1989; Lehman, 1989) resulting, in part, from a U.S.-Israeli conference on elder abuse that took place in Israel (Wolf & Bergman, 1989). Similar to the U.S., research on elder abuse in Israel has increased in the 1990s (Neikrug & Ronen, 1993; Kerem, 1991/1992; Zoabi, 1995; Lowenstein, 1995; Lowenstein & Ron, 1999). These earlier Israeli studies, like many of those in the U.S., were based upon lay or professional perceptions of the problem; findings on family caregiving burden were extrapolated to the (likely) existence of elder abuse, and were limited to small samples living in a particular locale. As true of such studies in the U.S., generalizations were made or inferred to all in the country.

Unlike the U.S., however, early work on elder abuse in Israel included empirical work on maltreatment within institutional, rather than community, settings (Lowenstein, 1999). Additionally, as these earlier Israeli studies included mainly Israeli Jews of Western European origins, generalizations made about the existence of elder abuse within the entire Jewish society in Israel can be questioned. Such studies failed to address non-Jewish populations in Israel. In a study by Sharon and Zoabi (1997), Israeli professionals were asked to report on the existence of abused elderly Arabs, and it was found that elderly Arabs were less likely to be abused than elderly Jews (although differences were not statistically significant). Elderly Arabs living in urban areas were more likely to be abused than those in rural areas.

The U.K. British awareness of elder abuse has been closely driven by the twists and turns of successive public approaches to social policy. Glendenning (1993) has noted a continuing use of a system of Public Inquiries, following the discovery of scandals of abuse in large institutions. Similar to Israel, institutional care was seen in Great Britain as the primary site of elder abuse throughout the post-war period. However, with the turn to a privatization of services and growth of community care in the late 1980s and early 1990s, attention turned to abuse within the family. This was in part a consequence of right-wing ideological concern with a supposed breakdown in family obligations to care and partly a testimony to the strength of the private care home owner's lobby (Biggs, 1996).

With a change to a more social democratic political environment, attention has been paid to monitoring and inter-professional collaboration, and to the publication of "No Secrets," a Department of Health (2002) report for the protection of vulnerable adults. Studies have been undertaken to examine the degree to which local authorities have set up systems to address abuse (Mathew et al., 2003). It would appear that while 94% of Local Authorities have appointed Adult Protection Officers, few had developed post-abuse support services. The change in policy to include elder protection under the wide banner of protecting vulnerable adults has yet to be critically assessed.

This combination of influences in the UK has resulted in a swing back to concern with institutional abuse, this time tempered by an overall awareness of the need to promote the inclusion of marginalized social groups such as older people. Despite a sudden growth in research funding for late-life issues, none of this money has gone, at the time of writing, to the study of elder abuse. This is not to say that helping professionals and academics have been idle in promoting awareness of the problem, and there are currently two pressure/lobby groups; the largest of which, "Action on Elder Abuse," has worked closely with successive governments.

MODELS FOR THE STUDY OF ELDER ABUSE

It is believed that researchers wishing to engage in cross-cultural or cross-national studies of elder abuse face many challenges. The first one, affecting both methodological and analytic issues, pertains to the conceptualization of studies. Such a challenge requires the identification of differences and similarities in elder abuse within different populations. Included are considerations with regard to definitions and frameworks.

Definitions. As earlier stated, even in the U.S. there are no agreed upon definitions of elder abuse. Some studies include only abuse in private community based homes that are perpetrated by family, friends, or neighbors. Other studies include maltreatment within long-term care facilities perpetrated by a staff member or self-abuse that does not include another person who is the abuser. The differing definitions of elder abuse, as found in the U.S. or within any other country, are compounded by the differing definitions of abuse between cultures and countries. Accordingly, there is a need to be culturally sensitive and not to invoke one's own definitions of abusive behavior.

Conceptual Models. In the search for conceptual models for cross-national study of elder abuse, the co-authors have concluded that the utilization of particular models for the cross-national study of elder abuse currently remain in the realm of discussion. Some models are comprehensive and would seem to have significant potential. Gelles and Straus (1979) sought to develop a comprehensive theoretical model for integrating different causes of violence in the family. They concluded that intra-family violence (which would include elder abuse) is so complex and occurs for so many reasons that a conceptual or theoretical model would be "utterly useless." In lieu of a theoretical model, they "remain convinced of the feasibility and desirability of a general systems approach" (p. 575).

A systems perspective, which identifies subsystems, may hold promise for the study of elder abuse. Indeed, a systems model for the analysis of intra-family or interpersonal adversity (and potentially for elder abuse in worldwide context) is not new to the social sciences. Garbarino (1977), extrapolating from Brofenbrenner's human ecological perspective (1974), used a systemic orientation to explain child abuse. This perspective for understanding abusive behavior focuses on the mutual adaptation of a person to the environment, conceives the environment topologically as an interactive set of systems with interaction of subsystems, focuses on the issue of the social habitability, and asserts the need to consider political, economic, and demographic factors in shaping the quality of life for family members. "These factors produce the developmental dynamic; there is no 'pure context-free' development" (Garbarino, 1977, p. 722). While such a model can be used to study such adversity within a society, it has not been used for cross-national purposes.

More recently, a multi-systemic perspective has been used to describe (and intervene in) juvenile delinquents and drug users (Henggeler et al., 1991; Henggeler, Melton, & Smith, 1992; Scherer et al., 1994). This framework includes three subsystems that can be used to explain elderly abuse and which might be helpful for the understanding of elder abuse in a cross-national perspective. The following is an extrapolation of the multi-systemic perspective applied to elder abuse. The first system focuses upon the *Physiologic Characteristics* of an abuser and includes attention to the propensity for abusive behavior (by virtue of aggressiveness, sensation seeking, and substance and drug addiction) and gender, perinatal issues, temperament, and cognitive factors, as well as a personality. A second subsystem is the *Familial Subsystem* within which can be found structural variables such as household composition and living arrangements, and the past style of parenting (which regard the development of adult children's personalities and needs which can lead to abusive behavior in later years), the development of attitudes and role modeling, the existence of family conflict or marital conflict, family patterns of role division, family norms, the status of the aged within the family, degree of family bonding, use of alcohol and drugs by family members, and past exposure to child and/or spouse abuse. Surrounding the Familial Subsystem is the larger *Contextual Subsystem* which includes consideration of peers, school or work settings, neighborhoods and communities, identity groups (for example, religion, social class, ethnicity), dominant and pervasive formal laws (with regard to the treatment of older or impaired persons), and informal social norms (regarding social attitudes toward aging and old age).

It appears that such systemic models may be useful for the study of elder abuse within a particular locale with a particular population, but may not lend itself to the cross-national study of elder abuse. This is due for several reasons including competing and conflicting definitions of elder abuse within and between countries, and multicultural groups being studied which are either without analytic differentiation or sampling controls. Clearly, more work and thought needs to go into the conceptualization of frameworks for the study of elder abuse in different countries and with different cultural groups.

Generalizations. In the search for commonalities in the development of cross-national studies on elder abuse, reliable and valid measurement instruments are imperative for use with populations not sharing common values, mores, and languages. Challenging the perceived contextual national character of elder abuse is the fact that the study of elder abuse cannot easily be measured by a common national "yardstick," for different subgroups exist within each nation having different as well as common values and norms.

As discussed for the U.S., UK, and Israel, any study purporting to report on elder abuse in a country without differentiating the population is subject to the scrutiny (if not criticism) of those who are sensitive to the diversity of subpopulations. National surveys produce aggregate, but undifferentiated, findings. More focused studies on elder abuse (that is, to a particular sub-sample) may result in a more conceptually meaningful sample, but a population more idiosyncratic than can be useful for: (1) comparisons with other sub-samples in a country, (2) national generalizations, or (3) international studies.

On the one hand, large-scale surveys of elder abuse produce data that can be assessed for general trends and for the comparison with large-scale studies from other countries. Obscured are the subgroup dynamics. On the other hand, however, more focused (and limited) studies might get closer to the causative relationships within a subculture but the specificity of such work might not lend itself to comparative analyses (or cross-cultural or international studies). Thus, there are important decisions to be made before pursuing the comparative analyses of elder abuse in different countries.

As has been suggested, it may be that the behavior toward family members (including the elderly) in a culture or society is considered normative, appropriate, and acceptable by that group, yet is viewed negatively as abusive by outside researchers. However, it may be the case that the definition of elder abuse in one county is the same as the definition of elder abuse in another.

Thus, there is a moral dilemma for the researcher, as well as for others. Classroom discussions in higher education have often considered the concept of "cultural relativity," whereby the ethnocentric criticism of behavior of people from another society is deemed to be insensitive to the unique features of the foreign society giving rise (and, perhaps, justification) to that behavior. Yet, professional groups (i.e., social workers, nurses, psychologists), although understanding the historical, economic, or cultural reasons for certain forms of adversity (i.e., child, spouse, elder abuse) within a population, may nonetheless invoke certain absolute moral standards for correct and incorrect treatment of people. This is to wonder whether the abuse of children, wives, or elderly persons can be justified by reasons of cultural relativity.

The elder abuse researcher involved in cross-cultural and cross-national studies may encounter colleagues from other countries who do not share similar definitions, standards, and values about interpersonal behavior. While those found within such countries as the U.S., UK, Israel, and Canada might be comparable, this may not be true for other countries.

CONCLUSIONS

This article represents an antecedent effort by the authors to identify and discuss the challenges that confront researchers wishing to engage in cross-national study of elder abuse. It is believed that findings from such studies will have importance not only for individual countries, but also for the discovery of the differences and commonalities in the abuse of elderly persons between nations and within nations. Hopefully, the result of such comparative studies will be the development of more sophisticated knowledge regarding the causes of elder abuse, as well as the sharing of different types of interventions which can focus upon the prevention of elder abuse as well as interventions after the occurrence of abuse.

Each case of elder abuse is different and occurs for many reasons, and is potentially influenced by the abuser's individual personality, family of origin, social class, race or ethnicity, religion or religiosity, age, and gender. Elder abuse takes place within different sub-cultural contexts which influences attitudes and values with regard to the elderly as well as the definition of different acts of commission and omission as right or wrong. Accordingly, cross-national conceptual models are needed for embracing such complexities while not projecting the values and definitions of abuse from any one country. The key here is to provide an orientation that is both generalizable and open to diversity.

The development of cross-national research models that can lead to furthering both heuristic knowledge of elder abuse and the development of programs and services await further developments on the construction of models that will incorporate the differing definitions of elder abuse for diverse populations within distinct societies. Without such models, cross-national studies of the abuse of older persons will either remain descriptive comparisons or may be criticized for being ethnocentric or not paying attention to the unique features of people from different ethnic, religious, or racial groups. The extrapolation of programs to combat elder abuse from one society to others, without consideration of differences in definitions, values, and populations, may result in inappropriate and ineffective actions.

This article does not address abuse perpetrated by two or more persons, multiple forms of abuse occurring either concurrently or consecutively to an individual, self-abuse, or within congregate settings by individuals paid to provide care. Attention has focused primarily upon abuse within community-based dwellings within which the abusers are members of the elder's support system. This adds further complexity for studying elder abuse within and between countries. Hopefully, such issues, and others, will be addressed in subsequent work that will have implications for elder abuse research and the development of programs and policies for the prevention of and intervention in the problem of elder abuse in different countries.

REFERENCES

Anetzberger, G., Korbin, J.E., & Tomita, S.K. (1996). Defining elder mistreatment in four ethnic groups across two generations. *Journal of cross-cultural gerontology* 11: 187-212.

Bennett, G., Kingston, P., & Penhale, B. (1997) *The dimensions of elder abuse*. London: Macmillan.

Biggs, S. (1996). Family concern: Elder abuse in British social policy. *Critical Social Policy*, 16.2:63-88.

Biggs, S. (2003). Elder abuse and social policy. Elder abuse: Can we achieve a world without violence? Unpublished presentation. Queen Sofia Center for Family Violence. Valencia, Spain.

Biggs, S., & Kingston, P. (1995). Special edition on elder abuse. *Social Work in Europe*, 2.3:1-33.

Biggs, S., Kingston, P., & Phillipson, C. (1996). *Elder abuse in perspective*. Buckinghamshire: Open University Press.

Bozinovski, S.D. (2000). Older self-neglecters: Interpersonal problems and the maintenance of self-continuity. *Journal of Elder Abuse & Neglect 12*(1): 37-56.

Brammer, A., & Biggs, S. (1998). Defining elder abuse. *Journal of Social Welfare & Family Law 20*(3): 285-305.

Bronfenbrenner, U. (1979). *The ecology of human development: Experiments by nature and design*. Cambridge, MA: Harvard University Press.

Calasanti, T.M. (1996). Incorporating diversity: Meaning, levels of research, and implications for theory. *Gerontologist 36*(2): 147-156.

Chan, H.T. (1985). *Report of elderly abuse at home in Hong Kong*. Hong Kong: Council of Social Services.

Connell, C.M., & Gibson, G.D. (1997). Racial, ethnic, and cultural differences in dementia caregiving: Review and analysis. *The Gerontologist 37*(3): 355-364.

Department of Health (2000). No secrets: Guidance on developing and implementing multi-agency policies and procedures to protect vulnerable adults from abuse. London: DOH. United Kingdom.

Dunn, P.F., & Sadler, P.M. (1993). Claim making about elder abuse in Australia. *Australian Journal of Gerontology 12*(4): 42-46.

Garbarino, J. (1977). The human ecology of child maltreatment: A conceptual model for research. *Journal of Marriage & the Family*, November: 721-735.

Gelles, R.J., & Straus, M.A. (1979). Determinants of violence in the family: Toward a theoretical integration. In Burr, W., Hill, R., Nye. F.I., and Reiss, I. (Eds.), *Contemporary theories about the family*. New York: The Free Press.

Glendenning, F. (1993). What is elder abuse? In Decalmer, P., & Glendenning, F. (Eds.), *The mistreatment of elderly people*. London: Sage.

Henggeler, S.W., Melton, G.B., & Smith, L.A. (1992). Family preservation using multisystemic therapy: An effective alternative to incarcerating serious juvenile offenders, *Journal of Consulting & Clinical Psychology 60*(6): 953-961.

Henggeler, S.W. et al. (1991). Effects of multisystemic therapy on drug use and abuse in serious juvenile offenders: A progress report from two outcome studies. *Family dynamics of addiction quarterly 1*(3): 40-51.

Hugonot, R. (1990). Abuse and violence against the elderly. *Bulletin de l'Academmie Nationale de Medecine 174*(6): 813-821.

Johansson, L. (1997). Support programs for caregivers: Some Swedish experiences. Unpublished paper presented at the 16th Congress of the International Association of Gerontology, Adelaide, Australia.

Johns, S., & Hydle, I. (1995). Norway: Weakness in welfare. *Journal of Elder Abuse & Neglect 6*(3/4): 139-156.

Kaneko, Y., & Yamada, Y. (1990). Wives and mothers-in-law: Potential for family conflict in post-war Japan. *Journal of Elder Abuse & Neglect 2*(1/2): 87-99.

Kerem. B.Z. (1991/92). Abuse of the helpless elderly. *Newsletter of the Israeli gerontological association*, No. 82 (Hebrew).

Kingston, P. (2003). Institutional indicators of elder abuse and neglect. Unpublished presentation. Elder abuse: Can we achieve a world without violence? Queen Sofia Center for Family Violence. Valencia, Spain.

Knudsen, D.D. (1992). *Child maltreatment: Emerging perspectives*. Dix Hills, NY: General Hall, Inc.

Kosberg, J.I. (1988). Preventing elder abuse: Identification of high risk factors prior to placement decisions. *The Gerontologist 28*(1): 43-50.

Kosberg, J.I., & Garcia, J.L. (Eds.). (1995). *Elder Abuse in international and cross-cultural perspective*. New York: The Haworth Press.

Kosberg, J.I., & Nahmiash, D. (1996). Characteristics of victims and perpetrators and milieus of abuse and neglect. *Abuse, neglect, and exploitation of older persons: Strategies for assessment and intervention*, L.A. Baumhover, & S.C. Beall, (Eds.), Baltimore: Health Professions Press, Inc.: 31-49.

Kosberg, J.I., & Kwan, A.Y.H. (1989). Elder abuse in Hong Kong and the United States: A comparative analysis with international implications. Unpublished paper presented at the Symposium on Cross-Cultural Perspectives on Elder Abuse, International Congress of Gerontology, Acapulco, Mexico.

Kozak, J.R., Elmslie, T., & Verson, J. (1995). Epidemiology of the abuse and neglect of seniors: A review of the national and international research literature. In M.J. MacLean (Ed.), *Abuse and neglect of older Canadians: Strategies for change*. Toronto: Thompson Educational Publishing, Inc.

Kwan, A.Y.-h. (1995). Elder abuse in Hong Kong: A new family problem for the Old East. *Journal of elder abuse: International and cross-cultural perspectives 6*(3/4): 65-80.

Lau, E.E., & Kosberg, J.I. (1979). Abuse of the elderly by informal care providers. *Aging* (September/October), 10-15.

Lawton, M.P., Moss, M., Fulcomer, M., & Kleban, M.H. (1982). A research and service oriented multilevel assessment instrument. *The Journals of Gerontology 37*, 91-99.

Lehman, H. (1989). Fraud and abuse of the elderly. In R.S. Wolf, & S. Berman (Eds.), *Stress, conflict, and abuse of the elderly*. JDC-Brookdale Monograph Series, Jerusalem.

Lowenstein, A. (1989). The elderly victim and the welfare services. *Stress, conflict and abuse of the elderly*, Wolf, R.S. & Bergman, S. (Eds.), Jerusalem: Brookdale Series, pp. 99-110.

Lowenstein, A. (1995). Elder abuse in a forming society: Israel. *Elder abuse in international and cross-cultural perspectives*, Kosberg, J.I., & Garcia, J.L. (Eds.), New York: The Haworth Press, Inc., pp. 81-100.

Lowenstein, A. (1999). Elder abuse in residential settings in Israel. *Journal of Elder Abuse & Neglect 10* (1/2): 133-152.

Lowenstein, A., & Ron, P. (1999). Tension and conflict factors in spousal abuse in second marriages of the widowed elderly. *Journal of Elder Abuse & Neglect 11*(1): 23-45.

Mathew, D., McReadie, C., Askham, J., Brown, H., & Kingston, P. (2002). The response to no secrets. *Journal of Adult Protection 4*(1): 1-12.

McCallum, J. (1993). Elder abuse: The new social problem? *Modern medicine of Australia.* September: 74-83.

Mui, A.C., & Burnette, D. (1994). Long-term care service use by frail elders: Is ethnicity a factor? *Gerontologist 34*(2): 190-198.

Neikrug, S.M., & Ronen, M. (1993). Elder abuse in Israel, *Journal of Elder Abuse & Neglect 5*(3): 1-19.

Ogg, J., & Munn-Giddings, C. (1993). Researching elder abuse, *Ageing and society 13*: 389-413.

Penhale, B. (2003). The concept of elder abuse: Breaking the silence. Unpublished presentation. Elder abuse: Can we achieve a world without violence? Queen Sofia Center for Family Violence. Valencia, Spain.

Pillemer, K. (1986). Risk factors in elder abuse: Results from a case control study. In K. Pillemer, & R.S. Wolf (Eds.), *Elder abuse: Conflict in the family* (pp. 239-263). Dover, MA: Auburn House.

Pillemer, K. (1988). Maltreatment of patients in nursing homes: Overview & research agenda. *Journal of Health & Social Behavior 29*(September): 227-238.

Pillemer, K., & Finkelhor, D. (1988). The prevalence of elder abuse: A random sample survey. *The Gerontologist 28*(1): 51-57.

Pillemer, K., & Moore, D.W. (1989). Abuse of patients in nursing homes: Findings from a staff survey. *The Gerontologist 29*: 314-320.

Rosenblatt, D.E. (1996). Documentation. In L.A. Baumhover, & S.C. Beall (Eds.), *Abuse, neglect, and exploitation of older persons* (pp. 145-161). Baltimore, MD: Health Professions Press.

Sanchez, Y.M. (1996). Distinguishing cultural expectations in assessment of financial exploitation, *Journal of Elder Abuse & Neglect 8*(2): 49-59.

Scherer, D.G., Brondino, M. J., Henggeler, S.W., Melton, G.B., & Hanley, J.H. (1994). Multisystemic family preservation therapy: Preliminary findings from a study of rural and minority serious adolescent offenders. *Journal of Emotional & Behavioral Disorders 2*(4): 198-206.

Shah, G., Veedon, R., & Vasi, S. (1995). Elder abuse in India. *Journal of Elder Abuse & Neglect 6*(3/4): 101-118.

Sharon, N., & Zoabi, S. (1997). Elder abuse in a land of tradition: The case of Israel's Arabs, *Journal of Elder Abuse & Neglect 8*(4): 43-58.

Shaw, W.S. et al. (1997). A cross-cultural validation of coping strategies and their associations with caregiving distress. *Gerontologist 37*(4): 490-504.

Shiamberg, L.B., & Gans, D. (1999). An ecological framework for contextual risk factors in elder abuse by adult children. *Journal of Elder Abuse & Neglect 11*(1): 79-103.

Smith, J.P. (1994). Measuring health and economic status of older adults in developing countries. *Gerontologist 34*(4): 491-496.

Soeda, A., & Araki, C. (1999). Elder abuse by daughters-in-law in Japan. *Journal of Elder Abuse & Neglect 11*(1): 47-58.

Tatara, T. (1993). Understanding the nature and scope of domestic elder abuse with the use of state aggregate data: Summaries of the key findings of a national survey of state APS and aging agencies. *Journal of Elder Abuse & Neglect 5*(4): 35-57.

Wolf, R.S., & Bergman, S. (1989). *Stress, conflict, and abuse of the elderly.* JDC-Brookdale Institute of Gerontology, Jerusalem.

World Health Organization/International Network for the Prevention of Elder Abuse (2002). Missing voices: Views of older persons on elder abuse. Geneva: WHO.

Zoabi, S. (1995). Elder abuse in the Arab society in Israel: Myth or reality. An MA Thesis. Haifa: Haifa University (in Hebrew).

A National Look at Elder Abuse Multidisciplinary Teams

Pamela B. Teaster, PhD
Lisa Nerenberg, MSW, MPH
Kim L. Stansbury, MSW

SUMMARY. Elder abuse multidisciplinary teams (MDTs) include professionals from diverse disciplines who work together to review cases of elder abuse and address systemic problems. Using an e-mail survey format, the authors received information from 31 MDT coordinators across the country representing fatality review teams, financial abuse specialist

---

Pamela B. Teaster is Vice President, National Committee for the Prevention of Elder Abuse and Assistant Professor, PhD Program in Gerontology, University of Kentucky School of Public Health, 306 Health Sciences Building, 900 South Limestone, University of Kentucky, Lexington, KY 40536-0200 (E-mail: pteaster@uky.edu). Lisa Nerenberg is Consultant, National Committee for the Prevention of Elder Abuse, 1906 Barton Street, Redwood City, CA 94061 (E-mail: lnerenberg@aol.com). Kim L. Stansbury is a Doctoral Candidate, PhD Program in Gerontology, 306 Health Sciences Building, 900 South Limestone, University of Kentucky, Lexington, KY 40536-0200 (E-mail: klstan2@uky.edu).

The authors wish to thank the representatives of the multidisciplinary teams for their dedication to addressing the problem of elder abuse and their assistance with this project.

A similar version of this article is under review by the partners of the National Center on Elder Abuse and the Administration on Aging.

[Haworth co-indexing entry note]: "A National Look at Elder Abuse Multidisciplinary Teams." Teaster, Pamela B., Lisa Nerenberg, and Kim L. Stansbury. Co-published simultaneously in *Journal of Elder Abuse & Neglect* (The Haworth Maltreatment & Trauma Press, an imprint of The Haworth Press, Inc.) Vol. 15, No. 3/4, 2003, pp. 91-107; and: *Elder Abuse: Selected Papers from the Prague World Congress on Family Violence* (ed: Elizabeth Podnieks, Jordan I. Kosberg, and Ariela Lowenstein) The Haworth Maltreatment & Trauma Press, an imprint of The Haworth Press, Inc., 2003, pp. 91-107. Single or multiple copies of this article are available for a fee from The Haworth Document Delivery Service [1-800-HAWORTH, 9:00 a.m. - 5:00 p.m. (EST). E-mail address: docdelivery@haworthpress.com].

teams, medically oriented teams, and "traditional" teams. The coordinators provided information on the functions their teams perform, the importance of specific functions, cases reviewed, composition of teams,
policies and procedures, administration, funding, and challenges to effective functioning. Teams expressed only mild concern for breaches in
confidentiality. MDTs stressed the importance of input by professionals
from the legal community for successful team functioning. *[Article copies available for a fee from The Haworth Document Delivery Service:
1-800-HAWORTH. E-mail address: <docdelivery@haworthpress.com> Website:
<http://www.HaworthPress.com> © 2003 by The Haworth Press, Inc. All rights
reserved.]*

KEYWORDS. Multidisciplinary team, elder abuse, interdisciplinary
team, financial abuse, fatality review, coordination

Multidisciplinary teams (MDTs), groups of professionals from diverse disciplines who come together to review abuse cases and address
systemic problems, are now a hallmark of elder abuse prevention programs. Teams first emerged in the early 1980s in recognition of the fact
that clinical and systemic issues that abuse cases frequently pose exceed
the boundaries of any single discipline or agency.

Teams are believed to offer many benefits to professionals, clients, and
communities. In addition to helping individual service providers resolve
difficult cases, the team review process has been credited with enhancing
service coordination by clarifying agencies' policies, procedures, and
roles and by identifying service gaps and breakdowns in coordination or
communication. Teams may also enhance members' professional skills
and knowledge by providing a forum for learning more about the strategies, resources, and approaches used by multiple disciplines.

The rapid proliferation of MDTs across the United States and Canada
in the last two decades has been accompanied by a growing demand for
highly specialized expertise in such areas as financial abuse, fatality review, and medical issues. Federal, state, and local governments have increasingly acknowledged the importance and benefits of MDTs and
have responded by providing resources, technical assistance, and statu-
tory authority.

Currently, there is a paucity of research examining elder abuse
MDTs. The research that does exist is localized, focuses on team development, and highlights the benefits of MDTs (Manitoba-Seniors-Direc-

torate, 1994; Wasylkewycz, 1993; Wolf, 1988). A recent article by Malks, Schmidt, and Austin (2002) deals specifically with a financial abuse specialist team in California. However, research does not address the functions and composition of MDTs and is not national in scope. Although anecdotal evidence suggests that teams offer tangible benefits to their members and communities, in-depth studies to identify how they function and demonstrate their impact on the problem of elder mistreatment have not been conducted. To begin to shed light on the functioning of teams, the National Committee for the Prevention of Elder Abuse (NCPEA), as partner in the National Center on Elder Abuse (NCEA), carried out a national survey. Team representatives were asked to identify key features of teams, explain variations, describe specialized teams, and identify common obstacles and how they are being addressed. The information presented below provides a picture of the various types of teams that responded to the survey. Further, it provides a framework for decision-making for groups that are considering starting teams or enhancing existing teams, and sets the stage for future research on teams' impact and effectiveness.

METHODS

Because no national list of MDTs was available, the authors requested the help of NCPEA's Board of Directors and subscribers to NCEA's list serve (operated by the American Bar Association's Commission on Law and Aging) to identify and suggest elder abuse teams. The request yielded approximately forty recommendations. The authors did not provide a specific definition of teams in order to capture a wide variety. However, they attempted to include teams that represented a diverse mix in terms of size of membership, focus, geographic location, and length of time in existence. The sample included "traditional" MDTs as well as specialized teams including financial abuse specialist teams (FASTs), teams with a medical orientation, and fatality review teams.

After approval by the University of Kentucky's Institutional Review Board, the authors sent e-mail letters to representatives or spokespersons of 40 teams. The e-mail communication explained the project, invited representatives of MDTs to participate, and advised potential participants of project timelines and processes. Thirty-two (32) team coordinators indicated their willingness to participate, and the project group sent out 32 surveys to them. Coordinators were given two weeks to complete the surveys and return them via e-mail, fax, or conventional mail. At the end of that period, members of the project group made follow-up calls to ensure the highest possible response rate. Of the original 40 team coordinators contacted, thirty-one returned surveys, for a response rate of 77.5%.

Data Collection Instrument

The survey instrument (Appendix A) was developed in consultation with members of NCPEA's Board of Directors and the project team to elicit information on defining features of teams such as sponsorship, funding sources, formalized policies and agreements, and membership. Respondents were also asked to identify challenges MDTs encountered as well as successful resolutions. They were further asked to describe products and accomplishments. Prior to sending the survey to the entire group, it was pilot tested with two team coordinators. The project group examined their responses and made inquiries regarding ease of completion. Suggestions that the project team deemed appropriate were then incorporated into the final survey that was sent to respondents.

Raw data were entered by a doctoral level graduate student in the PhD Program in Gerontology at the University of Kentucky and cross-checked for accuracy with the assistance of another doctoral level gerontology student. The doctoral level assistant contacted respondents for clarification when questions arose regarding the information provided on the survey. Data were analyzed by faculty and graduate students at the University of Kentucky using descriptive statistics.

RESULTS

Functions of Teams

To identify the most frequently performed functions of MDTs, respondents were given a checklist and asked to indicate those they perform. They were also invited to add additional functions.

The two most frequently cited functions of teams (Table 1) were providing expert consultation to service providers and identifying service gaps and systems problems (93.5% each). Nearly all teams also update new members about services, programs, and legislation (90.3%). Well over three-fourths of teams perform the following additional functions

TABLE 1. Functions of the Team

Functions	Number of Respondents	%
Providing expert consultation to service providers	29	93.5
Identifying service gaps and systems problems	29	93.5
Updating members about new services, programs, legislation	28	90.3
Advocating for change	26	83.9
Planning and carrying out training events	26	83.9
Planning and carrying out coordinated investigations or care planning	25	80.6

advocating for change; planning and carrying out training events; and planning and carrying out coordinated investigations or care planning.

Respondents were given the opportunity to list additional functions and added the following: providing training to team members on techniques, developing a coordinated community response to older victims of domestic violence and elder abuse victims, encouraging the investigation and prosecution of elder abuse crimes, resolving difficult health and social problems, cutting through delays that are built into "the system," and providing an opportunity for colleagues to offer support and advice on such issues as setting boundaries with clients and counter-transference.

Importance of Team Functions

In addition to identifying frequently performed functions, respondents were asked to rate the importance of each function on a one to five scale (with one being of no importance and five being essential). The highest ranking function was "providing expert consultation to service providers," which was rated as "Very Important" or "Essential" by 71% of respondents (Table 2).

Approximately half the teams ranked as "Very Important" or "Essential" the following functions: updating members about new services, programs, and legislation; identifying service gaps or systems problems; planning and carrying out coordinated investigations or care planning; and carrying out training events. As was the case with the earlier question, respondents were invited to list additional functions and to indicate their importance. Ranked as "Essential" were providing training to team members on techniques, developing a coordinated community

TABLE 2. Teams' Ranking of Functions as Very Important/Essential

Functions	Number of Respondents	%
Providing expert consultation to service providers	22	71.0
Updating members about new services, programs, legislation	18	58.1
Identifying service gaps and system problems	17	54.9
Planning and carrying out coordinated investigations or care planning	16	51.6
Planning and carrying out training events	14	45.2
Advocating for change	11	35.5

response to older victims of domestic violence and elder abuse victims, and encouraging investigation and prosecution of elder abuse crimes.

Types of Cases Reviewed

Most MDTs conduct case reviews, but they may handle the review process quite differently. For example, some teams review all types of elder abuse cases, while others focus on certain types. Nearly three-fourths (71.0%) review cases involving all types of abuse and neglect. Seven teams (22.6%) focus on financial abuse cases. Of these, five described themselves as Financial Abuse Specialist Teams (FASTs), a model developed in Los Angeles in the early 1990s and since replicated in other communities. Despite the common name, there are wide variations among the FASTs. For example, one FAST meets every two weeks, only includes representatives from public agencies, and places an emphasis on its rapid response to deter abuse and preserve assets. Another FAST has over 50 members, includes representatives from many private, non-profit agencies, and meets quarterly.

One team in the sample identified itself as a "fatality review team," a model that was originally developed in the fields of child abuse and domestic violence to review suspicious deaths or "near-deaths." Five additional teams indicated that they review fatalities but did not specifically call themselves fatality review teams. Two teams focused on medical issues in cases involving clients with multiple medical problems or cognitive decline.

Several teams indicated that they focus on particularly problematic cases, such as self-neglect cases, cases involving persons with mental illness and mental retardation, high-risk situations, and cases in which guardianship is being considered. Although many of the teams address systemic problems and issues, two teams indicated that they focus exclusively on systemic issues (as opposed to clinical issues related to client care).

Team Attendance

Respondents were asked to indicate how many people regularly attend team meetings. The question was posed in this way (as opposed to asking for number of members) because teams that operate informally may welcome all interested professionals to attend and do not require them to sign membership agreements. Nearly one-half (45.2%) of the teams have an average attendance of between five and 10 people. Just over one-quarter (25.8%) routinely have between 10 and 20 participants, nearly one-tenth (9.7%) have between 20 and 30 people attend regularly, and nearly one-tenth (9.7%) routinely draw more than 30 participants. One team typically has fewer than four in attendance (3.2%). Two teams did not respond to the question (6.5%).

Attendance Requirements. A fourth of MDTs (25.8) require members to attend a certain number of meetings yearly (e.g., five to ten). Three teams indicated that missing a certain number of meetings (e.g., three consecutive meetings) is grounds for dismissal. Typically, team members are encouraged to provide alternative attendees in their absence if they are unable to attend.

Frequency of Meetings. Nearly three-fourths of MDTs (74.2%) meet monthly (9.7% meet every two weeks, 9.7% meet every other month and 3.2% meet quarterly). One Team (3.2%) meets as needed in addition to its regularly scheduled meetings. To streamline meetings, some teams have structured agendas, which include such items as introductions, reviews of confidentiality, guest speakers or educational presentations, and updates on services or developments in the field.

Categories of Membership

MDTs were asked specific questions about their members. Teams reported that they recruit individual members, invite agencies to join and to designate representatives, or both. Individual members participate for their own benefit and represent their own viewpoints or perspectives, while agency members may serve as liaisons between their organizations and the team, convey agency policy and perspectives, and commit resources. Well over one-half of the teams (64.5%) allow individuals to join regardless of agency affiliation.

Organization members include private non-profit agencies, public agencies, and for-profit agencies (including professionals in private practice). Some teams only permit non-profit agencies and individuals who work for non-profit agencies (61.3%) to join. Slightly over one-third (35.5%) permit for-profit businesses to participate. Two teams only include representatives from public agencies.

Certain teams have created special categories of membership. For example, some have "core member" (e.g., Adult Protective Service, known as APS, or law enforcement), categories that must be filled at all times, and other categories that are considered desirable but not required. Teams may extend certain benefits to some members and not others, including the right to present case. Over one-half (58.1%) permit any team member to present cases, while others (29.0%) only allow certain members to do so (one team only permits APS workers to present cases, and another permits APS, Ombudsmen, law enforcement, and private attorneys to present). Still, others (25.8%) allow any service provider in the community to present cases, regardless of whether or not they are members.

Respondents indicated that the responsibilities of members also vary. For example, some teams require certain members to provide additional consultation or training between meetings and another uses "technical advisors" who do not routinely attend meetings but who are called upon for assistance as needed.

Disciplines Represented

Respondents were asked to indicate what professional disciplines are represented on their teams (Table 3). The most commonly cited were police and sheriffs, which was listed by 93.5% of respondents. APS workers participate on 83.9% of teams. Disciplines included on more than half of the teams are: providers of geriatric mental health services, prosecutors, aging service providers, public guardians, and domestic violence advocates. Other disciplines represented on fewer than 50% of teams include nurses, physicians, non-geriatric mental health professionals, and victim-witness advocates. Approximately one-third (32.3%) include representatives from financial institutions, and another one-third (32.3%) include clergy. Approximately over one-quarter (25.8%) include retired professionals.

TABLE 3. Professionals Represented on Teams

Disciplines	Number of Respondents	%
Police/Sheriff	29	93.5
Adult Protection Services	26	83.9
Geriatric Mental Health Services	25	80.6
Prosecuters	22	71.0
Aging Service Providers/Public Guardians	20	64.5
Domestic Violence Advocates	16	51.6
Nurses	15	48.4
Physicians	13	41.9
Non-Geriatric Mental Health Professional	13	41.9
Victim-Witness Advocates	13	41.9
Representatives from Financial Institutions	10	32.3
Clergy	10	32.3
Retired Professionals	8	25.8

Respondents were invited to list other disciplines and service categories included on their teams, and over one-half (51.6%) did so. These included ethicists, animal care and control officers, public administrators, probation and parole personnel, code enforcement personnel, resource specialists, firefighters, a retired judge, housing managers, housing advocates, personnel from assisted living facilities, members of public utility boards, in-home service providers, realtors, representatives from state long-term care licensing and regulatory agencies, hospital social workers, emergency medical personnel, providers of services for persons with developmental disabilities, media representatives, homeless shelter staff, health department personnel, health statistics specialists, health advocates, and certified public accountants.

Level of Team Formality

Respondents were asked several questions about formalized policies and procedures they employ and written materials they use to document or support policies and procedures, including meeting summaries, memoranda of understanding, "job descriptions" for members, orientation materials, policy and procedures manuals, and membership categories. These are described below (Table 4).

TABLE 4. Level of Team Formality

Method	Number of Respondents	%
Summarized Proceedings	17	54.8
Contracts/Memoranda of Understanding	16	51.6
Case Review Guidelines	16	51.6
Policy and Procedures Manuals	10	32.3
Job Descriptions	9	29.0
Orientation Manuals	9	29.0
Term Limits	7	22.6

Proceedings of Meetings. Over one-half (54.8%) of MDTs produce written records of meetings, which may be in the form of "minutes," summaries of the proceedings or case reviews, and recommendations. One team uses *genograms* to graphically depict the content of the team review (charts that graphically describe the social and familial relationships between individuals, a technique primarily used by mental health professionals to help identify positive and negative influences affecting an individual).

Teams that produce written records of meetings vary in how they use and disseminate them. Over one-half (51.6%) disseminate information on case reviews to team members and others. One MDT disseminates minutes to members but excludes information on case reviews, while another sends minutes to non-members in addition to members (including all police departments in the county, the district attorney, the Sheriff's Department, state adult protection, the public administrator, and a legal center for handicapped and older adults) as a way to educate these groups about the issue. A medical team includes case review summaries in clients' medical charts. One team that produces minutes keeps them in a special team book maintained by the program coordinator, who provides summaries upon request.

Contracts and Memoranda of Understanding. Just over one-half (51.6%) of MDTs require members to sign contracts or memoranda of understanding, which typically include provisions for confidentiality and terms of membership. Over one-fourth of teams (29.0%) require agency supervisors or administrators to sign contracts or memoranda of understanding, affirming the agencies' commitment to assign representatives and to replace representatives who are unable to meet their commitments.

Guidelines for Review of Cases. Just over one-half (51.6%) of teams use case review guidelines to provide direction or suggestions to presenters on what information to include in case presentations and the order in which to present it. Typically included are the client's living arrangement, support network, functional status, a description of the abuse and/or other presenting problems, and a history of attempted interventions or services.

Policies and Procedures Manuals. Approximately one-third (32.3%) of teams indicated that they have formal policies and procedures manuals. Only one team keeps the manual on disk rather than having it in hard copy due to the sensitive nature of its contents.

Job Descriptions. Over one-fourth (29.0%) use job descriptions for members, which may be contained in membership agreements, member handbooks, or elsewhere. The state of Wisconsin has developed a manual for its counties that includes job descriptions for representatives from the fields of law enforcement, medicine, law, domestic violence, financial management and mental health, as well as clergy. In addition to outlining the specific duties and responsibilities of each representative, Wisconsin's job descriptions also contain detailed requirements with respect to education, experience, training, knowledge, skills, and abilities. For example, it is recommended that law enforcement representatives have associates' degrees in criminal justice or another social science.

Orientation Materials. Approximately one-fourth of teams (29.0%) use orientation materials, which usually include handbooks that contain general information on elder abuse, pertinent laws, research articles, policies, mission statements, confidentiality agreements, by-laws, etc. One team has produced a video that all new members must view.

Term Limits. Nearly one-fourth (22.6%) of the teams have term limits for members, the most common of which is one year. The majority of teams (77.4%) allow members to serve more than one term. An annual renewal process may serve as an opportunity to review members' participation during the year and determine whether they have met their obligations to the MDT.

Other Information. Other written materials used by teams include a handbook for coordinators and written protocols. Some teams solicit input from members through routine or occasional surveys that ask how useful meetings are to members or by requesting suggestions for educational presentations. They may further ask members to provide information about case outcomes (e.g., were prosecutions successful as a result of team interventions; were assets or property recovered and, if so, what was the amount). Team members may be asked to indicate how many hours they have contributed during and between meetings and to estimate their associated *pro bono* contributions. Some teams ask members to fill out feedback forms at the end of every meeting.

Administration

MDTs were asked to provide information about administration. Four teams (12.9%) were coordinated by an Area Agency on Aging, and APS administered 10 (52.6%) teams. Other arrangements included administration by a district attorney's office or in collaboration with agencies/organizations such as a university, a local non-profit, or sheriff's office. Some operate informally without designated administrators. Activities associated with team administration that were cited included producing and sending out agendas, meeting announcements and minutes; arranging for meeting space; recruiting members and negotiating contracts and memoranda of understanding; preparing materials such as handbooks and job descriptions; producing and disseminating minutes; selecting cases; serving as a focal point for questions; and, in the case of some teams, following up on members' recommendations.

Leadership

Adult Protective Services (APS), the agencies mandated to respond to reports of abuse, neglect, and exploitation of older adults in most states, play a prominent role in MDTs. Nearly one-third of teams (32.3%) are administered by APS programs alone or in collaboration with other agencies (e.g., one team involves collaboration between APS and a hospital-based geriatric program). Following APS, Area Agencies on Aging (AAAs) (12.9%) are the next most likely entity to administer teams. Just over one-half (51.6%) of the teams surveyed are administered by other agencies. These include a county attorney's office, a private non-profit agency, a state attorney general's office, a university, and an "elder abuse provider" agency.

Funding and In-Kind Support

MDTs were asked to describe their sources of funding and in-kind support. The most common source of support to teams is APS programs, which provide support to 38.7% of the teams surveyed. Most APS support is in-kind (92.0%), which includes staff time (this may be for case workers, supervisors, support and clerical staff), meeting space, and the printing and mailing of materials. One-fourth of APS programs (25.0%) provide funding, with amounts ranging from $70 to $250.

Area Agencies on Aging (AAA) are the second most common source, providing support to 32.3% of the teams (again, most support is in-kind). Monetary support from AAAs includes elder abuse funds authorized under the Older Americans Act. Dollar amounts ranged from $3,000 to $85,122 annually.

Nearly one-half of MDTs (48.4%) receive support from other sources. Monetary support is provided by a state department of public safety, a state justice assistance council, the American Association of Retired Persons (AARP), and foundations. Funding amounts from these sources ranged from $500 to $10,000 yearly. Sources of additional in-kind support included an attorney general's office, a college of medicine, a county hospital district, a state attorney, providers of mental health and medical services, law enforcement, and a medical examiner's office.

Calculating the costs of operating a team was complicated by the fact that few teams have dedicated staffing. Staffing tasks are often shared by several individuals, are likely to fluctuate over time, and may be carried out intermittently and in concert with other tasks. Comparing costs was further complicated by the fact that teams engage in such diverse activities as community outreach, professional training, and research, all of which require very different levels of support. In addition, those that rely on in-kind support typically do not track costs. Consequently, teams' responses to questions about their costs varied widely, with some stating that there were no costs associated with the team, with one team indicating that it operates on an annual budget of over $85,000. Other MDTs were unable to respond to the question.

Sources of Technical Assistance

Teams receive guidance and technical assistance from a variety of sources, the most common of which is state agencies. State units on aging, state APS programs, and offices of attorneys general provide assistance to approximately one-third (32.3%) of the teams surveyed. These agencies provide manuals, sample materials, and training. Examples include the Illinois Department of Aging, which creates resource materials, brochures, posters, and videos. Other sources of technical assistance include national organizations

(9.7%), such as NCPEA, which operates a program of local affili-
ates, and a statewide coalition of teams.

Challenges

MDTs have encountered numerous challenges. Respondents were
asked to provide information about these challenges and to describe the
initiatives they have taken to address them (Table 5).

Lack of Participation by Certain Disciplines. Approximately one-half
(48.4%) of the teams indicated that they experienced difficulty gaining or
maintaining participation by certain disciplines. Foremost among these
was law enforcement (42.9%). Other underrepresented disciplines include medical professionals, clergy, prosecutors, attorneys, representatives from financial institutions, providers of services to young disabled
adults, pharmacists, state long-term care licensing and regulatory agencies, county attorney's offices, and mental health workers.

Maintaining an Adequate Number of Cases. Nearly one-fourth of
teams (22.6%) indicated that they have trouble finding enough cases to
present. One reason cited was that APS staff members are too busy to prepare case summaries. In addition, many communities now have more
than one team, which creates "competition" for cases. Teams have attempted to increase the number and diversity of cases by sending out
e-mail reminders about meetings and, in communities with more than one
team, clarifying the types of cases reviewed by each.

Confidentiality. Although the researchers had anticipated that breaches
in confidentiality would be a major concern of teams, only four respondents (12.9%) indicated that this was a challenge for them. Respondents
were also asked to indicate if they had, in fact, experienced breaches.

TABLE 5. Challenges That Teams Face

Challenges	Number of Respondents	%
Lack of Participation by Certain Disciplines	15	48.4
Maintaining an Adequate Number of Cases	7	22.6
Failure of Certain Groups to Present Cases	5	16.1
Confidentiality	4	12.9
Animosity Among Members	3	9.7
Failure to Agreed Upon Follow-Through	3	9.7
Members' Feeling Time Is Not Well Spent	2	6.7

Only one team reported experiencing a "close call." This relatively moderate level of concern may reflect teams' satisfaction with measures they have taken to preserve confidentiality.

Measures that MDTs have taken to ensure confidentiality included confidentiality agreements, which are employed by well over one-half (64.5%) of the teams and the use of pseudonyms or initials when discussing cases (48.4%). Over one-third of teams (35.5%) operate in states that have special laws that permit the sharing of information and/or immunity laws, which protect information disclosed at meetings from being used as evidence in civil actions or disciplinary proceedings. Other methods for ensuring confidentiality included written reminders about confidentiality (with applicable state code sections) on monthly meeting agendas, outlining confidentiality provisions in a memorandum of understanding members sign when they join the team, and not disseminating case summaries. One respondent observed that as teams gain experience and members get to know each other, concerns about confidentiality have decreased.

Other Challenges. Other challenges cited included the failure of certain groups to present cases (16.1%), animosity among members (9.7%), failure of members to follow through on actions to which they have agreed (9.7%), and members not feeling their time is well spent (6.7%). Additional challenges cited by single respondents included: Agency representatives delegated to attend meetings do not have the authority needed to make systems changes, and those with the authority do not attend, lack of funding and support, and failure to achieve "buy-in" from members whose participation is not voluntary (e.g., they are mandated to participate).

Tangible Products

In addition to case reviews, teams engage in many other activities, the most common being those related to training (58.1%). Training materials produced by teams include booklets, packets, manuals, PowerPoint presentations, and a curriculum and workbook. Groups targeted for training include bank employees, clergy, gatekeepers, the public, law enforcement, medical students and practitioners, and mandated reporters. Training events include conferences, workshops and "train-the-trainer programs." Topics covered in training sessions include fraud prevention, medical issues, APS and its role in receiving reports (including services offered, who must report, and what to expect once a case has been assigned to APS for investigation and follow-up), how to recognize and investigate fiduciary abuse, real estate fraud, and how to gather evidence of incapacity for guardianships and lawsuits.

Approximately one-third of MDTs (32.3%) produce other materials (not related to training) including brochures, laminated law enforcement cards that list elder abuse statutes, resource cards for law enforcement, a video on victim impact, a video on FAST, websites, annual reports, newsletters, resource guides, public service announcements, and handbooks. Replication materials produced by teams include videos and how-to manuals.

Other activities and accomplishments cited by respondents included the development of interagency agreements (25.8%), legislation (19.4%), a protocol for law enforcement, and referral guidelines for APS workers. One team was developing a volunteer program to recruit retired bank personnel to assist in investigating financial abuse cases. The program is patterned after a successful model developed in Oregon.

CONCLUSIONS

This study was a first effort to shed light on the role, processes, varieties and accomplishments of MDTs on a national level. Although limited in sample size (it did not study the hundreds of teams that have emerged nationwide in the last two decades), it underscores the benefits and costs of teams, highlights trends, and provides insight into the challenges teams face. Further, it reveals some of the difficulties program planners and policy makers address in anticipating the direct and indirect costs of operating teams.

Several findings are noteworthy. Assisting workers resolve difficult abuse cases is frequently cited as the primary goal of teams and is why some teams were initiated. Although this function was rated as the most important performed by teams, the overwhelming majority of teams also identify service gaps and update members about new services, resources, and legislation. This finding suggests that, although case reviews are important in themselves, as previously believed, they frequently reveal systemic problems and point to the need for new services, resources, legislation, and information about new resources and developments.

Also noteworthy is the importance of legal expertise and input on teams. Police and sheriffs, prosecutors and public guardians are among the six most commonly included disciplines represented on teams, surpassing such groups as medical professionals and domestic violence advocates.

The relatively mild concern for breaches in confidentiality was also surprising in light of anecdotal evidence to suggest otherwise. One example is a situation wherein a fatality review team in California refrained from reviewing cases until the state passed legislation that permitted the sharing of information.

Reported costs of operating teams varied widely, with some teams clearly not knowing their true operational costs, although it was obvious that costs were incurred. It may be that teams should examine, through systematic outcome evaluation, their true costs and benefits at regular intervals to determine whether they meet their operational goals or whether such goals can be reasonably achieved.

In conclusion, MDTs play a key role in communities' response to elder abuse and are highly valued by those who participate. Among the benefits they cited were strengthening community relationships, eliminating or ameliorating turf wars, promoting team work and cooperation, providing assistance on cases referred for guardianship, helping clients secure improved medical care, and enhancing members' understanding of services. Clearly, the strength of MDTs is their ability to mobilize professionals from a wide range of disciplines to confront the complex and growing problem of elder mistreatment.

REFERENCES

Malks, B., Schmidt, C.M., & Austin, J. (2002). Elder abuse prevention: A case study of the Santa Clara County financial abuse specialist team (FAST) program. *Journal of Gerontological Social Work, 39*, 23-40.

Manitoba-Seniors-Directorate. (February 1994). Abuse of the elderly: A manual for the development of multidisciplinary teams. *MDT Working Group on Elder Abuse, Winnipeg, Canada.*

Wasylkewycz, M.N. (1993). Elder Abuse Resource Centre, a coordinated community response to elder abuse: One Canadian perspective. *Journal of Elder Abuse & Neglect, 5*, 21-33.

Wolf, R. S. (1988). Elder abuse: Ten years later. *Journal of the American Geriatrics Society, 36*, 758-762.

A Forensic Medical Examination Form for Improved Documentation and Prosecution of Elder Abuse

Diana Koin, MD

SUMMARY. A new innovative tool for improved elder abuse documentation and prosecution has been developed in California. Created by a cross-disciplinary group of elder abuse experts, the form provides a format for thorough evaluation of the multiple forms of abuse as well as guiding the examiner through both physical and psychological findings. The form is in two parts. The first part provides systematic documentation of basic demographic information, a checklist to document the victim's concurrent forms of abuse, assessment of independent function,

Diana Koin is Director, Elder and Dependent Adult Abuse Education, California Medical Training Center, University of California Davis Medical Center, University of California Davis Health System, FSSB Building, 4800 Second Avenue, Suite 2200, Sacramento, CA 95817 (E-mail: diana.koin@ucdmc.ucdavis.edu).

The author wishes to thank all members of the Forensic Medical Report: Elder/Dependent Adult Abuse and Neglect development committee for their creativity, compassion, and dedication.

This project was funded by a grant from the California Governor's Office of Criminal Justice Planning.

Medicine, law enforcement, social services, and prosecution were part of the team that created the form. A draft version of the form was then distributed to health care, social services, and law enforcement personnel for final comment and critique.

[Haworth co-indexing entry note]: "A Forensic Medical Examination Form for Improved Documentation and Prosecution of Elder Abuse." Koin, Diana. Co-published simultaneously in *Journal of Elder Abuse & Neglect* (The Haworth Maltreatment & Trauma Press, an imprint of The Haworth Press, Inc.) Vol. 15, No. 3/4, 2003, pp. 109-119; and: *Elder Abuse: Selected Papers from the Prague World Congress on Family Violence* (ed: Elizabeth Podnieks, Jordan I. Kosberg, and Ariela Lowenstein) The Haworth Maltreatment & Trauma Press, an imprint of The Haworth Press, Inc., 2003, pp. 109-119. Single or multiple copies of this article are available for a fee from The Haworth Document Delivery Service [1-800-HAWORTH, 9:00 a.m. - 5:00 p.m. (EST). E-mail address: docdelivery@haworthpress.com].

and cognitive screening. The second part leads the examiner to describe the physical status of the patient and to document all injuries on body diagrams. *[Article copies available for a fee from The Haworth Document Delivery Service: 1-800-HAWORTH. E-mail address: <docdelivery@haworthpress.com> Website: <http://www.HaworthPress.com> © 2003 by The Haworth Press, Inc. All rights reserved.]*

KEYWORDS. Forensic, abuse, neglect, justice, protocol

Lack of reliable medical documentation of elder abuse and neglect has been an ongoing detriment to successful prosecution of these cases. Information is often cursory, inconsistent, and incomplete. Although injuries may be documented in the patient's medical record, they are not recorded in a routine and specific fashion that would enable law enforcement and prosecutors to readily locate the critical pieces of information.

Other forms of interpersonal violence have had success with forensic documentation of injuries. Utilization of a state-wide form for documentation of injuries and evidence collection in California has grown in acceptance in child abuse and sexual assault (Peterson, 2002).

The elder abuse victim is often traumatized by the events unfolding at the time the crime is identified. The forensic examination will enable physicians to focus on many aspects of the patient. A thorough approach will provide reassurance and comfort to the victim.

This paper describes the development of a forensic examination tool for elder and dependent adult abuse. Although the form described was created to specifically meet the legal requirements of elder abuse law in California, the strategies inherent in a forensic approach to elder abuse have universal applicability. Although multiple tools for elder abuse assessment exist (Fulmer, Guadagno, Dyer, and Connolly, 2004), a forensic method will provide important new strategies for improving prosecution.

THE LEGISLATIVE MANDATE

The California Legislature passed Senate Bill 502 in 2001. Entitled "An act to add Section 11161.2 to the Penal Code, relating to domestic violence and elder and dependent adult abuse and neglect, and making an appropriation therefore," it gave direction to develop forensic examination forms. Senator Deborah Ortiz has long championed bills that improve the status of victims of interpersonal violence. Because of her prior experience, she was willing to introduce legislation directing the creation of forensic forms for domestic violence and abuse of elders and dependent adults. The forms would amplify the one page mandated reporting form that health care providers in California are mandated to complete. The intent of the legislation was to create a form that would provide for comprehensive forensic examination. Injuries and neglect would be documented. Reliable information about a victim's functional and cognitive status would be obtained.

Senator Ortiz' staff sought suggestions from constituencies with significant interest in the field, with particular emphasis on health care providers and the criminal justice system. Organizations participating in early discussions of a forensic form included the California Medical Association, the California District Attorneys Association, the California Sheriff's Association, Department of Social Services, and the California Department of Justice.

The Governor's Office of Criminal Justice Planning selected The California Medical Training Center (CMTC), a special family violence education project at the University of California Medical School at Davis, to facilitate development of the forms for domestic violence and elder and dependent adult abuse. The designation of the CMTC as the organization responsible for providing leadership for development of the form added continuity to existing forensic forms for reporting of interpersonal violence. Its leadership had previously led the committees that developed the state's forensic reporting forms for sexual assault and child sexual assault, as well as providing trainings throughout the state on how to use the forms.

The bill succinctly identifies the rationale for development of a forensic medical examination reporting form:

> The Legislature finds and declares that adequate protection of victims of domestic violence and elder and dependent adult abuse has been hampered by lack of consistent and comprehensive medical examinations. Enhancing examination procedures, documentation, and evidence collection will improve investigation and prosecution efforts.

The legislation does not identify a funding mechanism for the examination.

FORM DEVELOPMENT: THE PROCESS

Experts in the field of abuse of elders and people with disabilities throughout California were invited to be members of the form development committee. Professionals with expertise in health care, law enforcement, social services, forensic technology, judiciary, and prosecution agreed to be part of the committee. Health care representation included physicians, nurses, and psychologists. In addition to academic physicians who are abuse experts, practitioners from primary care and emergency medicine participated.

The initial draft was based on California's sexual assault forensic reporting form that has wide acceptance throughout the state. Although the committee was given free reign to create an entirely different form, the decision was made to maintain a similar format. Familiarity would enable health care providers already completing forms for other crimes of interpersonal violence a rapid transition to the elder abuse form.

Committee members brought to the task special knowledge and expertise in abuse and neglect of elders and people with disabilities. Representation was sought to include not only health care providers but also professionals from the criminal justice system. Law enforcement, judicial, prosecution, forensics, and probate court representatives provided invaluable input to the process, offering balance to the health care perspective. The nursing representatives offered both gerontological and emergency room expertise. The participating physicians had backgrounds in geriatric medicine, emergency medicine, primary care, and developmental disabilities. Social service committee members represented Adult Protective Services and a member with wide spread training and development expertise. One of the psychologists on the committee has expertise in both clinical assessment and a special interest in capacity issues whereas the other psychologist has extensive law enforcement experience.

Committee members had specific tasks to accomplish. Prior to the meeting, participants were asked to review existing forensic forms for sexual assault and child abuse, read the legislation establishing the development of the form, and to bring with them any other forensic medical assessment tools that they utilized in their own work, or that they could obtain from colleagues. The logistics of the committee's work and the statewide review process of the form were established. In parallel with the sexual assault and child abuse forms, the elder and dependent adult abuse form would be accompanied by a detailed set of instructions and a protocol providing background materials and guidelines.

ISSUES AND CONTROVERSIES

The committee found several areas controversial as they worked together on the form. Issues were raised by both committee members and colleagues in the field. Although not formalized, consensus was used as the strategy for decision-making. Agreement was often reached when a problem was analyzed in terms of providing the most reliable evidence for prosecutors. At times, colleagues who were not members of the committee but were aware that the form was under development also offered comments and suggestions.

One of the issues of intense debate was the location where the forensic examination should be performed and the appropriate strategy for using the form. Although the committee envisioned possible circumstances where the examination would take place in a primary care setting or even possibly a nursing home, a hospital emergency room with forensic familiarity was felt to be the appropriate setting. An emergency department was the location most likely to be able to collect and process evidence reliably. Nonetheless, as the state of California has a vast array of community needs, varying from large urban centers with tertiary health care to remote rural areas with minimal medical presence, the goal was to create a form useful throughout the state.

Throughout the committee's meetings, discussion ensued about who would complete the form. The earliest version of the form had two parts, the first being for specially trained nurses and social workers, and the second section being completed by physicians after examining the victim. Later, the separation between different providers completing part one or part two was removed from the form, only to be reinstated in the final versions of the form. In the final nine-page form, part one will be health professionals who have completed elder abuse forensic training; part two will be completed by physicians, physician assistants, nurse practitioners, and assault-specialist nurses.

Decisions about demographic data to be collected received a great deal of focus by the committee. Pillemer (2000) pointed out that "Research on elder abuse has been inconsistent due to the sources of data on the problem." Although not the primary role of the form, utilization of a forensic form throughout the state would facilitate data collection. California has a paucity of reliable elder abuse and dependent adult abuse criminal justice data. While not an initial goal of the project, a central data collection site would provide important information about volume and trends in the field.

Perhaps the most controversial area of the form was what should be done to assess cognitive ability. The committee concurred that there was great need for the victim's mental status to be documented in the form, but members had lengthy discussions about the best strategy to accomplish this goal. Cognitive screening is important in abuse and neglect cases because it identifies victims' levels of dependency and vulnerability. Dementia is highly associated with risk of abuse (Dyer, Pavlik, and Murphy, 2000). After lengthy debate, the committee selected the Mini-Mental State Examination (Folstein, Folstein, and McHugh, 1975) as the tool for documenting cognitive status. Although it is limited in that it is intended only to be a screening test and that it has recognized educational and cultural bias, the committee felt that it is the mental status assessment that is most widely used and recognized. Consent for a forensic examination is documented on the form and a large print version will accompany the form. The protocol to be distributed to examiners elaborates fundamental rationale and standards of consent. The protocol also details the differences between mandated reporting (required of all health care providers in California) and forensic examination, which is optional. The goal of forensic examination is to gather evidence and document pertinent findings that will likely lead to prosecution. However, in the anticipated trainings for examiners it will be emphasized that forensic examination is to be performed in a manner that will be an intervention leading to enhanced safety and well-being for the victim. Examiners will also be trained to clarify to victims the confidential nature of the examination and to explain that only legal recipients will be given the information. For persons lacking capacity to provide consent themselves, a surrogate decision maker's signature is included on the form. The committee had concerns that the surrogate decision maker may well be the perpetrator, but it was suggested that if the surrogate refused the consent to examination that the instructions on the form would recommend consultation with the local district attorney's office and the court system. Thus in some situations, the consent would be provided by a court-appointed temporary conservator. In addition to the victim's agreement to consent for the examination, his or her signature is required to document that they have been informed about possible restitution from the Victims of Crime fund.

The prosecutor serving on the form development committee wanted identification of "Great Bodily Injury" on the form. Great Bodily Injury is the legal description of injuries severe enough to lead to felony prosecution and to increase the severity of punishment to the perpetrators. Discussion about inclusion of a separate section that would enable prosecutors to easily identify injuries of that severity was requested. One of the benefits of including a specific section would have been the potential for education of health professionals about the necessity of careful documentation of those kinds of injuries. However, after meeting together it was decided to eliminate Great Bodily Injuries as an identified section for fear that some health providers would not complete it and thus imply that no "Great Bodily Injury" had taken place. Instead, the section of the form devoted to describing abuse on body diagrams leads the physician to consider whether or not the victim has injuries of that severity.

The most controversial area for the committee was the length of the examination form. As the form is not mandatory, a time-consuming form might deter wide spread acceptance. The committee recognized that it was going to be difficult to enthuse emergency room physicians and specialized assault nurses about the superiority of the form if it took several hours to complete. The committee felt that there was actually a positive part in the length of the form, namely that by being comprehensive initially at the time of examination, physicians would feel assured that they had all of the relevant data necessary for court testimony later. This anticipated balancing-act between time versus future court adequacy was monitored informally in settings where the form was pilot tested. Pilot examiners told the committee that the examination time diminished with increased familiarity with the form and its comprehensiveness was reassuring when the case moved forward for prosecution. Inclusion of such things as mental status screening and functional assessment has been recognized as critically important. Sanders (2000) points out that one of the distinguishing characteristics of elder abuse is that it includes "issues of cognitive impairment and decision-making capacity, functional ability, comorbid conditions, and financial dependency." One of the difficulties inherent in the field of elder abuse is the multiplicity and complexity of the crimes. This factor, too, dictated a comprehensive form that would be inclusive of the many forms of abuse and neglect of elders and people with disabilities.

Innovations to the field were contributed during the course of development of the form. The second page of the form is a comprehensive elder abuse check list covering all the forms of abuse mandated for reporting in California: physical, neglect, self-neglect, sexual, abandonment, financial, abduction, and isolation. Psychological abuse is also included although it is not mandated in the state so that there will be documentation in the future that a victim was intimidated, threatened, or harassed. The committee recognized that health care providers would focus on physical abuse, and sought a strategy for expanding the examiner's appreciation of the multiplicity of potential concurrent crimes. Thus, the check list will serve as a reminder to provide an expanded examination for all types of abuse.

Committee members discussed the fact that legal proceedings for abuse and neglect cases may poorly reflect the gravity of a victim's actual experience at the time of the abuse. One of the most important factors that may fail to be recorded or documented is the patient's actual degree of pain and suffering. The form includes both a place for noting a patient's reported physical pain (from one to ten) and also offers the smiling-to-sad faces for the victim to choose his or her level of pain if it is verbally difficult to articulate the severity of his or her discomfort.

Evidence collection is critical, and the form guides the examiner in gathering physical evidence. The examiner is directed about not only how to collect evidence, but how to label it and to assure that its' handling fulfills appropriate chain-of-custody guidelines. It is anticipated that some physicians completing a forensic examination of abused elders will have little experience with criminal evidence. The form will provide guidance for the examiner to assure reliable collection of forensic evidence. The importance of this was described by Thomas (2000), "Effective case building in the emerging field of elder abuse and neglect must have effective forensic medical evidence."

THE DRAFT REVIEW PROCESS

Once the draft form was finalized to the satisfaction of the form development committee, it was sent throughout the state of California for review and comment. As the elder and dependent adult abuse form was completed concurrently with the new form for domestic violence forensic reporting, the two forms were mailed together. An attempt was made to ask for review from all parties and organizations with knowledge and expertise in elder abuse and dependent adult abuse throughout the state. This included all hospitals, law enforcement, adult protective services, ombudsmen, and professional organizations of those likely to encounter elder and dependent adult abuse victims. More than four thousand copies of the draft form were distributed throughout the state, and reviewers were invited to return their comments via mail, fax, or electronic mail. More than two hundred responses were returned. Although this represented a five percent return rate, reviewers provided thoughtful and lengthy critique of the form. Reviewers identified concerns ranging from format issues to substantive concerns about clarity.

A subcommittee of the form development committee reviewed all comments about the form. Suggestions that were readily incorporated were added to the next version of the form immediately. Some comments were viewed as being beyond the scope of the project; they were forwarded for review by the form development committee as a whole. All substantive critique was also reviewed by the committee.

The form development committee met to review the comments obtained from the state-wide review and to finalize the form. Because the most consistent criticism was about the length of the form (nineteen people said the form was too long; one said the form was too brief) a careful review ensued to make certain that all eight pages of the form were deemed necessary. No change was made in the length of the form.

ANTICIPATED OUTCOMES

Education will be undertaken state-wide to train health care providers how to correctly complete the Forensic Medical Report: Elder/Dependent Adult Abuse and Neglect. The goal of the trainings will be to develop a corps of skilled elder abuse forensic examiners working throughout the state of California. The California Medical Training Center will also be developing a more advanced level of forensic specialist: an elder abuse forensic medical expert. In addition to being skilled at interpretation of forensic findings, the expert will implement quality assurance leadership to assure standardization of the examinations.

Physician training will be focused on forensic examination and evidence collection. As the form utilizes body diagrams with legends describing multiple possible lesions and injuries, physicians will have hands-on practical sessions to maximize successful training outcomes. Skill stations will be utilized to focus the participant on specific forensic issues, such as evidence collection, injury identification and diagrams, malnutrition assessment, and pressure ulcer staging and documentation. The inclusion of a module of the California Medical Training Center's Forensic Photodocumentation Course will introduce physicians to the importance of capturing evidence visually. Training will include discussion of the interface between medicine and the criminal justice system, enabling physicians to understand the key role they can play in successful prosecution. Case presentations will be utilized to accomplish this, and will offer doctors the opportunity to learn how forensic evidence collection and documentation may be the deciding factor in cases where victims have suffered great bodily injury. Throughout the training, physicians will be encouraged to recognize that careful forensic examination and documentation will provide them with the best chance to avoid appearing in court because their report is complete enough to stand alone or to fully succeed as witnesses.

Because part one of the form is be completed by doctors, physician extenders, nurses, and social service providers, trainings will include all likely participants. All trainees will learn how to best utilize the elder abuse checklist to enhance their ability to identify multiple concurrent forms of abuse. Functional assessment will be taught utilizing mini-case studies regarding victims with limited abilities to perform activities of daily living and instrumental activities of daily living. Examiners will gain experience in the correct way to administer a mini-mental state examination. The implications of diminished functional ability or cognitive capability for risk of physical abuse, neglect, and financial abuse will be underscored.

Although not a specific expectation of the original legislation, the Forensic Medical Examination Form has the potential of providing exceptional data. The data could be used for improved demographic analysis, establishing patterns of forensic injury, documentation of the concurrence of the multiple crimes of abuse, and serve as a baseline for outcome studies of interventions.

REFERENCES

California Senate Bill 502, Chapter 579 (2001). An act to add Section 11161.2 to the Penal Code, relating to domestic violence and elder and dependent adult abuse and neglect.

Dyer, C.B., Pavlik, V.N., Murphy, K.P. (2000). The high prevalence of depression and dementia in elder abuse or neglect. *Journal of American Geriatric Society* 48, 205-208.

Folstein, M.F., Folstein, S., McHugh, P.R. (1975). Mini-Mental State: A practical method for grading the cognitive state of patients for the clinicians. *Journal of Psychological Research* 12(3), 189-198.

Fulmer, T., Guadagno, L., Dyer, B.D., Connolly M.T. (2004). Progress in elder abuse screening and assessment instruments. *Journal of American Geriatrics Society* 52, 297-304.

Peterson, M.P. (2002, June 28). California Medical Training Center (CMTC): Developing Forensic Medical Examiner Programs. *Unsilenced from Survival to Success, A*

Quarterly Sexual Assault Prosecution Newsletter by the California District Attorneys Association, 2(4), 1-5.

Pillemer, K. (2000, October 18). Critical Research Needs in the Study of Elder Abuse. *Elder Justice: Medical Forensic Issues Concerning Abuse and Neglect.* Washington, DC.

Sanders, A. B. (2000, October 18). Elder Justice Roundtable: An Emergency Room Perspective. *Elder Justice: Medical Forensic Issues Concerning Abuse and Neglect.* Washington, D.C.

Thomas, R. W. (2000, October 18). Elder Abuse and Neglect: Forensic Medical Evidence. *Elder Justice: Medical Forensic Issues Concerning Abuse and Neglect.* Washington, DC.

Elder Abuse Awareness in Faith Communities: Findings from a Canadian Pilot Study

Elizabeth Podnieks, EdD, RN
Sue Wilson, PhD

SUMMARY. Faith communities can play a critical role in the prevention of elder abuse and neglect by fostering heightened public awareness of elder mistreatment, as well as providing services to abused elders in the community. Faith leaders are among the most likely groups of caregivers to encounter cases of elder abuse, but unfortunately not all are aware of ways of identifying and effectively dealing with abuse. Religious leaders require training to educate them about elder abuse issues to identify the important roles they can play in prevention, intervention and treatment. Pastoral workers and theology students should also be exposed to educational concepts regarding this problem. In an age of ecumenism and interfaith movements, religious leaders must become a

---

Elizabeth Podnieks is affiliated with Ryerson University, School of Nursing 222 College Street, Toronto, Ontario M5T 3J1 (E-mail: onpea.info@utoronto.ca). Sue Wilson is affiliated with Ryerson University, KHS-241-Y, 350 Victoria Street, Toronto, Ontario, M5B 2K3 (E-mail: suwilson@ryerson.ca).

The authors acknowledge the contribution of research assistants Jessica Burnett and Alysa Golden.

[Haworth co-indexing entry note]: "Elder Abuse Awareness in Faith Communities: Findings from a Canadian Pilot Study." Podnieks, Elizabeth, and Sue Wilson. Co-published simultaneously in *Journal of Elder Abuse & Neglect* (The Haworth Maltreatment & Trauma Press, an imprint of The Haworth Press, Inc.) Vol. 15, No. 3/4, 2003, pp. 121-135; and: *Elder Abuse: Selected Papers from the Prague World Congress on Family Violence* (ed: Elizabeth Podnieks, Jordan I. Kosberg, and Ariela Lowenstein) The Haworth Maltreatment & Trauma Press, an imprint of The Haworth Press, Inc., 2003, pp. 121-135. Single or multiple copies of this article are available for a fee from The Haworth Document Delivery Service [1-800-HAWORTH, 9:00 a.m. - 5:00 p.m. (EST). E-mail address: docdelivery@haworthpress.com].

121

conduit for the well-being and safety of older adults. This paper dis-
cusses exploratory work undertaken in Ontario, funded by Health Canada (Ontario Region), the Ontario Trillium Foundation, and Justice
Canada to begin to uncover the extent to which faith leaders are aware of
instances of elder abuse, and what they might see as their role in addressing such problems in their faith communities. A thorough literature review suggests that while considerable attention has been paid to the
issue of elder abuse, researchers have not focused on the role of faith
leaders in addressing this complex problem. *[Article copies available for a
fee from The Haworth Document Delivery Service: 1-800-HAWORTH. E-mail
address: <docdelivery@haworthpress.com> Website: <http://www.Haworth
Press.com>* © 2003 by The Haworth Press, Inc. All rights reserved.]

KEYWORDS. Elder abuse, faith leaders, faith communities, prevention, education

INTRODUCTION

*"There is a reluctance to preach against abuse . . . The pulpit is not be-
ing used as effectively as it should be"* (focus group participant).

The abuse and neglect of older people occurs worldwide although it
is largely a hidden problem. The 1999 Canadian General Social Survey
asked Canadians about their experience of abuse. Seven percent of seniors reported some sort of emotional, physical, or financial abuse in the
five years prior to the survey (Dauvergne, 2003). Emotional abuse was
the most common form reported. Police reports from 2000 show that assault is the most common offence experienced by seniors, perpetrated
by family members. "Among those senior homicides committed by
family members between 1974 and 2000, spouses were the most likely
perpetrators (39%), followed by adult children (37%), and extended
family members (24%)" (Dauvergne, 2003:13). Sixty-eight percent of
seniors who were physically abused said that they were assaulted by a
family member. The abuser was more often an adult child than a spouse.
Male seniors were more likely than females to suffer financial or emotional abuse (Statistics Canada, 2000). As the proportion of seniors increases, so does the challenge of addressing the problem of abuse and
neglect of older persons.

Faith leaders may be an important key in the identification, intervention, and ultimate prevention of elder abuse. Older Canadians make up a

disproportionate share of those who identify with a faith tradition and attend churches, synagogues, or mosques. An Ontario study of the shelter needs of older Canadian women, found that older women would seek help from a place of worship if they experienced abuse. Thirty-three percent of respondents under the age of 76 identified a place of worship, compared with 52% of those over 76-years-old. This study was conducted in 1998 by the Ontario based Older Women's Network (OWN). Results are based on a survey of 106 women in 15 different languages, in five communities across Ontario.

LITERATURE REVIEW

Studies documenting the extent of elder abuse (McDaniel & Gee, 1993; McDonald & Collins, 2000; Pottie Bunge, 2000) have addressed a wide range of factors, including incidence, reporting, demographics, risk factors, intervention strategies, best practice models, and the limitations of existing resources. However, the idea that faith communities and faith leaders might be pivotal in responding to elder abuse has not been addressed by researchers. An American edited collection of works entitled *Abuse and Religion: When Praying Isn't Enough* (Horton and Williamson, 1988), and the landmark Canadian book by Nason-Clark (1997), *The Battered Wife: How Christians Confront Family Violence*, are two exceptions although both books look at family violence generally, rather than elder abuse. No references connecting faith or religious leaders or faith or religious communities to elder abuse were found in a literature search using Medline, CINAHL, and Academic Search Elite.

Certainly, a case has been made that Christian churches *should* proactively address issues of elder abuse (Nason-Clark, 1997; Eugene, 1995). Family violence experts such as Pagelow (1988), and other leaders in the area of religious issues affecting seniors such as Weaver and Koenig (1997) have clearly emphasized the need for all faith leaders to be proactive regarding their treatment of elder abuse. Faith leaders are in a unique position in their ability to identify, assess, and intervene in abusive situations because they see older people in their own context, over time, and have ongoing access to the senior's place of residence (Boyajian, 1991). However, we do not know how faith leaders feel about this role.

In their book *Abuse and Religion: When Praying Isn't Enough*, Horton and Williamson (1988) argued that clergy may hold certain attitudes about women's roles, duties, and vows of commitment that can influence how they respond to reports of abuse. According to Horton and Williamson, many North American women who seek help from faith leaders are often disappointed by the response of the faith leaders. In their study of 350 battered women, Pagelow and Johnson (1988), noted that 28% of the women reported seeking the help of local clergy. According to the women, the clergy responded by reminding them of their marital responsibilities, and advised them to forgive and forget. Clergy either suggested avoiding church involvement, or offered advice based on religious doctrine rather than the women's own needs. Another study of 1,000 battered wives from across the United States revealed that one-third of the women sampled had sought help from faith leaders. These women however, rated the effectiveness of the clergy as lower than most other formal supports (Bowker, 1988).

Nason-Clark (1997), asked ministers to estimate the percentage of married couples, in Canada, and within their own congregations who have experienced violence as part of their relationships. Ministers estimated that violence occurred in more than one-fourth of married couples (28.8%) in Canada, compared to estimates of less than one in five violent marriages (18.8%) in their own congregations. Ministers therefore, appeared to underestimate violent behaviour within their own pastoral charge. Further research is needed to determine whether these figures can be related to perceptions of elder abuse as well.

Some studies have focused on elder abuse within a specific cultural, but not religious, community (Brown, 1989; Griffin, 1994; Longres, 1992; Tattara, 1997; Knopf, Nackerud & Gorokhovski, 1999). Some of these may inform our understanding of elder abuse in faith communities. One study examined the perceptions that Korean-American elders held about elder abuse, taking into account both cultural and non-cultural influences (Cheung & Moon, 1997). From the elders' perspective, the problems associated with the abuse were due to a lack of respect, care, and sensitivity towards older persons' feelings and needs. The breakdown of 'Hyo' (the traditional parent-child relationship) was understood to foster the existence of abuse.

Korean elders suggested that mediators could help the family members share and understand the difficulties, expectations, disappointments, and misunderstandings between generations. Mediators could also potentially assess their circumstances, and generate specific plans to improve intergenerational treatment. The researchers suggested that the Korean-American community (including churches), could mitigate and prevent elder abuse and neglect by instituting programs that promote interactions and improve relationships between elderly parents and their adult children's families. The emphasis here is on building natural filial relationships, instead of removing them, to prevent further abuse.

The paucity of studies that look at elder abuse in religious communities speaks to the presence of a significant gap in our understanding of elder abuse. This pilot study begins to explore the notion that religious communities can play an integral role in the prevention and treatment of elder abuse. We have noted above that a high percentage of older women have said that they would seek help from their place of worship if experiencing abuse (Older Women's Network, 1998). Unfortunately, religious communities are rarely included as resources in training, education, prevention, or treatment literature. The absence of faith leaders and religious organizations in existing resource directories reinforces their lack of involvement in this problem, and suggest that this an important social support for seniors is not well tapped.

This study and its companion (published in this issue) asked faith leaders about their awareness of elder abuse, their responses to elder abuse in their faith communities, and their needs regarding information, education and resources to identify and respond to elder abuse. This study is based on qualitative open-ended individual and group interviews with twenty-one faith leaders and parish nurses in Toronto, Canada. The companion study is based on structured interviews with forty-nine faith leaders in Ontario, Canada. Together they provide insight into the ways faith leaders respond to elder abuse, the barriers they experience and the supports they seek.

THE STUDY

The project, "Raising Awareness of Elder Abuse in Faith Communities," started in 1999 to study the perceptions of–and responses to–elder abuse in faith communities in Ontario, Canada. The primary goal of the project was to increase the awareness of elder abuse among faith leaders, their congregants, and the public at large. The objective of the project was to develop and disseminate the strategies, supports, information and materials, and other activities to educate and empower faith leaders, religious communities, and congregants (including children and youth) on the issue of elder abuse. The present study and its companion are two pieces of the larger puzzle. This study was designed to solicit the views of a range of faith leaders to determine the extent to which they possess the necessary will, information and skills to be effective first contacts for elderly abused parishioners.

A strong coalition was formed to guide the research that included the sponsoring organizations of: Ryerson University Office of Research Services, the Older Women's Network (OWN), Women in Interfaith Dialogue/The League for Human Rights B'nai Brith Canada, University of Toronto Faculty of Social Work, and the Ontario Network for the Prevention of Elder Abuse. Clearly there are many people and agencies that realize the importance of a comprehensive study on this issue.

Initially, faith leaders representing a range of religious organizations were contacted in late 1999 and early 2000. In addition, members of the advisory board and community contacts were asked to refer faith leaders who might be willing to participate in an hour-long interview on the subject of elder abuse. Scheduling time with faith leaders was far more challenging than anticipated, as their discretionary time was often interrupted by unexpected needs of community members. Gaining their participation was therefore, very difficult and the sample size, was unfortunately small even for an exploratory study. In total there were twenty-one interviews. Sixteen participants were interviewed individually, and five were part of a focus group. Respondents included two rabbis, one Islamic Muslim lay leader, and three parish nurses. The rest of the participants were Christian, but eight of the interviewees represented diverse ethnic communities. While far from a representative sample, the twenty-one faith leaders and parish nurses represent Canada's main religious groups. According to the 2001 census, 43.2% of Canadians indicated their religious affiliation as Roman Catholic; 29.2% were Protestant, and 10.2% belonged to other religious groups. Over 16% of Canadians said they had no religious affiliation in 2001 (Statistics Canada, 2003, 18). In the interviews, faith leaders were asked about their perceptions of elder abuse, their responses to situations involving abuse of community members, barriers to confronting abusive situations and the kinds of materials they would find helpful in more effectively deal with elder abuse in their communities.

RESULTS

Perceptions of Elder Abuse Among Faith Leaders

Faith leaders identified a range of abuse, including physical, emotional, financial, and verbal abuse from husbands, wives, children, and caregivers both inside and outside of institutions. They provided a number of specific instances of abuse, including examples of elderly people being forced into nursing homes. The most comprehensive definition of elder abuse came from one faith leader who said, " Elder abuse is behavior that denigrates the dignity or infringes upon the personal liberties of the elderly." Neglect was thought to be the most prevalent form of abuse and the root of mental health problems such as Alzheimer's and dementia, as well as "heartsickness" and getting "sick to death." All faith leaders had a general understanding of the nature of elder abuse, but all tended to downplay the extent of abuse in their own religious communities.

Responses of Faith Leaders to Elder Abuse

All of the faith leaders interviewed for this study indicated that they were involved in advocacy regarding elder abuse, including talking to family members or convening staff meetings at nursing homes. However, they typically do not get involved in counseling members who have experienced abuse. Faith leaders in this sample have offered spiritual counseling, but not counseling around abuse. Instead, most choose to refer their parishioners to trained counselors within their faith community, including nuns or ethno-specific social workers. For example, the Muslim community has a Social Welfare Board, where social workers have the specific responsibility for seniors' issues. One faith leader explained that his credo is, "Thou shalt not kill," meaning that one must examine an allegation of abuse very carefully so as not to "kill" the reputation of an alleged abuser who may be innocent of wrongdoing. One clergy expressed reluctance to become involved with abuse or indeed with elderly parishioners. "My bishop said to me that he believes it is a ministry of reluctance. A lot of clergy do not like ministering to the elderly whether it is in institutions or at home." Only one faith leader talked about active prevention of elder abuse. In this case the community was planning a senior's home adjacent to the religious buildings so as to cut down on senior's isolation and therefore reduce instances of neglect. None of the participants indicated that they had ever contacted the police in a case of abuse.

In some faith communities, parish nurses provide holistic nursing services to members. The role of the parish nurse is to promote health and wellness in the body, mind, and spirit of the congregation (Ebersole, 2000). This could reasonably be expanded to include working with the clergy to intervene in cases of elder abuse. Parish nurses are welcomed into the homes of their clients, they are able to observe signs and symptoms of neglect, and most importantly they are trusted by both older persons and their families. There is a growing body of literature on parish nurses and further research is needed to examine the role of the parish nurse in working with other members of the faith community to prevent elder abuse and neglect.

Faith Leaders' Perceptions of Barriers to Supporting Elders Experiencing Abuse

Barriers to helping abused older adults were identified on two levels: The barriers to the older adult seeking help, and the barriers to the faith leader providing help. Several faith leaders mentioned that the effects of the abuse, such as isolation, dependency, mental and physical illness, could also prevent older adults from disclosing abuse. They also believed that older adults might be reluctant to report the violence because they had grown up in situations where abuse was not discussed. One faith leader referred to the older adults in his church as being intensely private; making it difficult for the clergy to know when to intervene and when to respect the desire for privacy among parishioners.

Participants also identified problems involving the stigma associated with abuse, and the potential for victim blaming as possible barriers to seniors. A number of faith leaders mentioned that the nature of the relationship between the faith leader and the older adult is also a complicating factor. Some thought that there would be no barriers to an elderly person who was practicing in his or her faith, because they would completely trust their religious institution. Most believed that the more the elderly congregant knew the religious leader, the more likely she or he would be to disclose the abuse. However, congregants are faced with barriers that are more specific to the church community. If the abuser and the abused are part of the same congregation, the faith leader may feel an obligation to both parties: "One parishioner is talking about another parishioner, who may or may not be a close blood relative, and who gets believed?" Another faith leader explained that "encouraging family members to uncover abuse on another family member's part is problematic because it turns family members against each other in the eyes of the church, even though abuse is involved." Another type of problem occurs when clergy have no contact with the elderly churchgoer's family. Although faith leaders expressed an obligation to follow up when they became aware of abuse, they were hesitant when they did not hear about the situation first hand. A parish nurse explained, "I worked in that area (older adult abuse), and people would go to their priest and it was taken very seriously, but the solution was to 'bear with it' . . . and that's something that needs to be talked about."

One priest who seemed to reflect the feeling of several faith leaders, spoke of the difficulty in addressing the issue of elder abuse in faith communities. He directly remarked, "I still think it's hard for people to name, and I think it's harder to do it in church." Another participant explained that in a culture that identifies strongly with the notion that "it is better to give than to receive," it is hard to feel empowered to say that one is not being cared for or neglected. Perhaps reflecting the patriarchal structure of most religious institutions, several mentioned that it was particularly hard for women to complain of abuse by family members, because they tended to blame themselves. To identify abuse is in effect saying, "My child or my niece or my nephew or somebody is really violating the Torah, the Bible."

One faith leader summed up the problem with the following observation: "I think that we've been somewhat reluctant to play an advocacy role and the parishioners seem reluctant to use the religious community as a resource for their family needs."

In many cases faith leaders lack the appropriate knowledge and intervention skills, and so are reluctant to become involved in abuse situations. One posed the question, "What if my level of awareness is not sufficient?" Many expressed the pressures they experience in serving members of their communities effectively: "We're there to help people in need and our tremendous emphasis on love and kindness and all of that, we as clergy, feel terribly guilty when we're not able to do these things and I don't know one member of the rabbinate who is good at being able to say, "Well, I would like to help, but . . ." According to another faith leader, the time pressures of religious services cut into the ability to engage in a social work role. "It is a heck of a lot more important to try to figure out how we're going to address abuse in the lives of our community than put fifty-seven hours into bazaar planning, which is the reason that people like me, feel we're really over-worked." When asked if clergy would be willing to attend a day-long conference and talk about some of these barriers and how to intervene in elder abuse issues, the response was lukewarm. One participant said, "I don't know, to go to a conference feels like you've really got to reorganize your life in a big way. However, to go to a half-day 'something or other' is a lot more doable." This response speaks to not just time restraints, but perhaps as well to the relative importance of the issue of elder abuse in faith communities in general.

Confidentiality is a concern for Catholic priests because of the role of the confessional. A Catholic faith leader acknowledged that elder abuse was brought to his attention (both by abusers and those being abused) during confession. When this happens, the priest is obliged to hold the information in strict confidence. This limits what could be disclosed to the interviewer in this study. Wicks (1996), observed that in North America considerable confusion exists over who actually owns and who can control the information a minister acquires and disseminates. Wicks' provocative discussion raised questions about whether or not the faith leader has an obligation to transfer the information that he or she has acquired in the area of counseling practices and confidential communications. In some cases, the law or professional standards suggest it belongs to the parishioner-client, in other cases to the faith leader, and in still others to society as a whole acting through its judiciary (Wicks, 1996: 40). Wicks postulates that the possibility of a charge of malpractice raises the question of ownership.

Faith leaders raised some concern regarding the public perception of the faith community: "Is this information going to make my community look as if its response to this problem is not sufficient?" It is important to all faith communities both to be doing what they can about the social problems within their communities, and to be seen as doing such. Some even asked, "What does the researcher think of how we are doing?"

While faith leaders seem to demonstrate a positive attitude regarding aging, pre-conceived notions of old age might prevent them from truly seeing the realities of the lives of their older followers. Shepard and Webber (1992), have noted that ageism, identified as one cause of the abuse of older adults, is almost as prevalent in local church congregations as it is in the general population. Negative stereotypes affect how older people view themselves and can contribute to their vulnerability to abuse. Filial piety and the cultural concept of the family may make it difficult for faith leaders to accept that older persons within their faith community are being abused. Boyajian (1991), pointed out that people in faith communities are inclined to think that elder abuse may possibly happen elsewhere, but not in their own communities. Abuse in ones own community is often invisible.

Resources and Training

The participants were initially asked what they thought would be helpful in the way of education for themselves, their elderly congregants and their community, on the issue of elder abuse. All agreed that it is very important to increase awareness of elder abuse. The interviewees thought that both the community at large and older members of religious communities could benefit from education or information sessions concerning elder abuse. Interestingly, materials aimed specifically at the religious leaders themselves were not mentioned in response to the initial question regarding needs. Perhaps this is because of the strong referral role most faith leaders take in response to elder abuse. It also may reflect the sentiment expressed in several ways that suggested that abuse is not a significant problem in *their* community–although they are aware of it existence elsewhere.

Nevertheless, faith leaders had several ideas about how best to inform seniors about the issue of elder abuse. These ideas included going into homes for the aged, attending social groups, and using newsletters to disseminate information. Accessing existing avenues as forums for social and educational purposes was strongly advised. All participants felt that resources must be developed in strict consultation with members of the community. All agreed that any materials developed must be culturally sensitive, and produced in the preferred language of the seniors. Some noted the importance of going beyond simple translation to create culturally relevant material. Others remarked that many seniors are isolated by language and for this reason, may be unable to, or feel uncomfortable about accessing services. Because faith communities are separated by language and philosophy, a joint initiative was seen as the most effective model. Individuals are presumed to be too time stressed to initiate something.

Interviewees from immigrant communities made the point that elder abuse is not necessarily a high priority in many immigrant communities. One stated, "Our community is solely preoccupied with finding employment and learning to speak English so that our members can survive in society." This sentiment was echoed by representatives from a number of communities including those with a long history of settlement in Canada. This point of view represents the thinking of community leaders, not those who experience abuse. However in the face of such an opinion, it is unlikely that solicitations for help regarding abuse would be taken seriously. Interestingly, representatives from non immigrant communities thought that the risk of abuse was higher in immigrant than non-immigrant communities where both elderly and caregivers are under enormous stress from isolation due to language and socio-economic barriers.

Religious leaders all talked about their lack of training in the issue of elder abuse, both at the seminary level and subsequent theological training. Training in the issue of elder abuse is extremely limited in seminaries, rabbinical schools and theological programs. One of the clergy in the focus group mentioned that a natural dissemination vehicle and opportunity for training may come in the form of seminars in "zones" or ministerial groups where clergy get together to explore and educate one another. Another participant mentioned that post-seminary programs would be a more effective vehicle for training because the "theological programs feel like they're always being asked to save the world and they're just trying to make sure that they can train a few people and get them out there."

The consensus among all of those interviewed was that more training is needed, but that it would be a hard to convince faith leaders to take time for training unless they had experienced the issue of elder abuse. Some faith leaders prefer to delegate, sending community affiliated designees to training or information sessions rather than attending themselves (Sheehan, 1989). This can make faith leaders a difficult group to target for training, particularly if the goal is to increase their knowledge about a particular topic, such as aging or elder abuse and neglect. Perhaps Nichols (1995), is right in suggesting that an important key to successfully targeting faith leaders for training is collaboration with community agencies. Indeed, one of the three most important factors that lead to the development of more aging programs within a faith institution is their collaboration with community agencies (Sheehan, Wilson, and Marella, 1988).

Self-education, participation in seminars, and the development of resources and strategies for the faith community as a whole are all ways to assist faith leaders to increase their knowledge of aging and elder abuse. When asked about preferred formats for educational materials, participants indicated a pamphlet and/or a video. One participant suggested a "best practice" guideline that would be "helpful for clergy in sort of wrestling with the problems and figuring out a way to do that so you're not betraying anyone in terms of your role as this person's faith leader." Role-playing or some sort of theatrical presentation was also cited as being a possible resource for effectively raising awareness of abuse issues.

Several faith leaders suggested "sermonettes" or homilies written by someone knowledgeable in the field of elder abuse so that the rabbi, priest, or other faith leader could deliver them. Case studies were also thought to be useful resources. These resources could be put together with other source material, to make a resource kit that the clergy could draw upon to raise awareness of the issue. The difference in preaching methodologies in different denominations or religious traditions was raised as a possible barrier to the utilization of such a resource. One participant said: "I think you're probably better, instead of planning one document, thinking of it with multiple quotations or multiple documents for different faith communities."

CONCLUSION

In Canada, as in most Western countries, the proportion of older adults in the population is increasing. This may mean that more seniors will be exposed to the risk of domestic abuse (Dauvergne, 2003: 10). Older people who suffer abuse and neglect are often reluctant to seek help. However, a trusting relationship between faithful older persons and their faith leaders may make disclosure of mistreatment more likely. An older adult may be less likely to fabricate a situation to a trusted clergy (Pagelow, 1988). Perhaps more than any other single resource, faith leaders are in the special position of being able to offer spiritual and emotional help and guidance to victims. Seniors should be able to view their faith community as a safe haven and place for spiritual renewal. In the face of abuse, the service of the church, temple or synagogue is a potential restorative source of support. The power of a higher spirit, the religious tradition of unconditional love and care are unique aspects of victim assistance that only a faith community can provide.

Despite the limitations of the study, the findings here suggest that faith communities may not be prepared to meet the needs of senior congregants, particularly their oldest members who, with advancing age, are at higher risk of abuse. Our findings suggest that appropriate materials and participation in educational sessions, may help faith leaders better respond to this growing population. The most effective means of identifying and combating elder abuse may well be a thorough understanding of the aging process. To this end, schools of theology and/or seminaries must seriously consider incorporating gerontology courses as part of their core curriculum for future faith leaders.

Faith leaders and community agencies must partner to ensure that spiritually sensitive social services are available to abused older adults. The work discussed in this paper is a step in that direction.

The information collected and disseminated through the project will inform and enlighten faith leaders, their communities, researchers, and policy makers of the role that faith institutions are, and should be, playing with respect to elder abuse. The more we can help the faith leader to improve and extend his or her ability to respond to abuse and neglect of older persons the more we will be helping the older, abused churchgoer.

REFERENCES

Bowker, L.H. (1988). Religious victims and their religious leaders: Services delivered to one thousand battered women by the clergy. *Abuse and Religion: When Praying Isn't Enough.* A.L. Horton, & J.A. Williamson (Eds.). Massachusetts, D.C. Health & Company.

Boyajian, J.A. (1991). *Elder Abuse: The view from the chancel in sexual assault and abuse: A handbook for clergy and religious professionals.* Pellauer, M.D., B. Chester, & J.A. Boyajian, (Eds). San Francisco, CA: Harper and Row.

Brown, A. (1989). A survey on elder abuse in one Native American tribe. *Journal of Elder Abuse & Neglect. 1* (2), 17-37.

Cheung, J., & Moon, A. (1997). Korean-American elderly's knowledge and perceptions of elder abuse: A qualitative analysis of cultural factors. *Journal of Multicultural Social Work.* 6 (1/2), 139-155.

Dauvergne, M. (2003). Family violence against seniors. *Canadian Social Trends.* Spring (68), 10-14.

Ebersole, P. (2000). Parish nurse leaders. *Geriatric Nursing,* 21(3), 148-149.

Eugene, J.R. (1995). A religious perspective. *Journal of Elder Abuse & Neglect,* 7(2-3), 157-175.

Griffin, L.W. (1994). Elder maltreatment among rural African Americans. *Journal of Aging & the Elderly,* 6(1), 1-27.

Horton, A. L., & J.A. Williamson, (1988). *Aging and Religion: When Praying Isn't Enough.* Massachusetts: D.C. Heath & Company.

Knopf, N., Nackerud, L., & Gorokhovski, I. (1999). Social work practice with older soviet immigrants. *Journal of Multicultural Social Work,* 7(1-2), 111-126.

Longres, J. (1992). Race and type of maltreatment in an elder abuse system. *Journal of Elder Abuse & Neglect.* 4(3), 61-83.

McDaniel, S.A., & Gee, E.M. (1993). Social policies regarding caregiving to elders: Canadian contradictions. *Journal of Aging & Social Policy.* 5 (1-2), 57-72.

McDonald, L., & Collins, A. (2000). Abuse and neglect of older adults: A discussion paper. *Ottawa: Health Canada. The National Clearinghouse on Family Violence,* 18-19.

Nason-Clark, N. (1997). *The Battered Wife: How Christians Confront Family Violence.* Louisville: Westminster John Knorr Press.

Nichols, A. (1995). Planning and implementing a state-wide collaborative gerontology education program for religious professionals in rural areas. *Journal of Religious Gerontology*, 9(2), 51-67.

Older Women's Network. (1998). *Study of Shelter Needs of Abused Older Women.* Toronto.

Pagelow, M.D. (1988). Abuse of the elderly in the home. *Abuse and Religion: When Praying Isn't Enough.* (pp. 29-37) A.L. Horton, & J.A. Williamson, (Eds.). Massachusetts: D. C. Heath and Company.

Pagelow, M.D., & Johnson, P. (1988). Abuse in the American Family: The Role of religion. *Abuse and Religion: When Praying Isn't Enough.* (pp. 1-11) A.L. Horton, & J.A. Williamson, (Eds.). Massachusetts: D. C. Heath and Company.

Pottie Bunge, V. (2000). Abuse of older adults by other family members. *Family Violence in Canada: A Statistical Profile, 2000.* V. Pottie Bunge, & D. Locke, (Eds.). Statistics Canada Catalogue No. 85-224.

Sheehan, N.W. (1989). The caregiver information project: A mechanism to assist religious leaders to help family caregivers. *The Gerontologist*, 29(5), 703-709.

Sheehan, N.W., Wilson, R., & Marella, L.M. (1988). The role of the church in providing services for the aging. *The Journal of Applied Gerontology*, 7(June), 240.

Shepard, G.H., & Webber, J.A. (1992). Life satisfaction and bias towards the aging: Attitudes of middle and older adult church members. *Journal of Religious Gerontology*, 8, 59-72.

Statistics Canada. (2003) Religions in Canada. Catalogue No. 96F0030XIE2001015. Ottawa: Minister of Industry.

Tattara, T. (1997). National conference on elder abuse. *National Conference on Understanding and Combating Elder Abuse in Minority Populations.* Notes.

Weaver, A.J., & Koenig, H.G. (1997b). Elder abuse: How to stop ignoring and start helping abused elderly. *Christian Ministry*, (July-August), 18-19.

Wicks, D.A. (1996). A minister's information-handling: Protections and constraints on a pastor's caregiving. *Journal of Religious & Theological Information*, 2(2), PG#s.

An Exploratory Study
of Responses to Elder Abuse
in Faith Communities

Elizabeth Podnieks, EdD, RN
Sue Wilson, PhD

SUMMARY. This study, conducted by Ryerson University, The Ontario Network for the Prevention of Elder Abuse, Older Women's Network, and the Centre for Applied Research (Faculty of Social Work, University of Toronto) examines faith leaders' perceptions of elder abuse, the actions taken by them in response to suspected or disclosed situations of elder abuse, and their knowledge and understanding of resources and services available for elder abuse intervention. Survey data was collected using an instrument that contained both open and closed-ended questions. The results of the study revealed that two-thirds of the clergy interviewed knew of, or suspected elder mistreatment among their parishioners. Faith leaders identified lack of education about elder mistreatment, lack of knowledge and/or skill in intervention

Elizabeth Podnieks is affiliated with Ryerson University, School of Nursing, 222 College Street, Toronto, Ontario M5T 3J1 (E-mal: onpea.info@utoronto.ca). Sue Wilson is affiliated with Ryerson University, KHS-241-Y, 350 Victoria Street, Toronto, Ontario M5B 2K3 (E-mail: suwilson@ryerson.ca).

The authors acknowledge the contribution of Joanne Daciuk and Lynn McDonald of the Centre for Applied Research, Faculty of Social Work, University of Toronto.

[Haworth co-indexing entry note]: "An Exploratory Study of Repsonses to Elder Abuse in Faith Communities." Podnieks, Elizabeth, and Sue Wilson. Co-published simultaneously in *Journal of Elder Abuse & Neglect* (The Haworth Maltreatment & Trauma Press, an imprint of The Haworth Press, Inc.) Vol. 15, No. 3/4, 2003, pp. 137-162; and: *Elder Abuse: Selected Papers from the Prague World Congress on Family Violence* (ed: Elizabeth Podnieks, Jordan I. Kosberg, and Ariela Lowenstein) The Haworth Maltreatment & Trauma Press, an imprint of The Haworth Press, Inc., 2003, pp. 137-162. Single or multiple copies of this article are available for a fee from The Haworth Document Delivery Service [1-800-HAWORTH, 9:00 a.m. - 5:00 p.m. (EST). E-mail address: docdelivery@haworthpress.com].

techniques and confidentiality issues as barriers to responding effectively to the abuse of elders. *[Article copies available for a fee from The
Haworth Document Delivery Service: 1-800-HAWORTH. E-mail address:
<docdelivery@haworthpress.com> Website: <http://www.HaworthPress.com>
© 2003 by The Haworth Press, Inc. All rights reserved.]*

KEYWORDS. Elder abuse, faith leaders, faith communities

INTRODUCTION

The issue of elder abuse has received increased attention by service
providers and researchers, although it remains publicly hidden for the
most part (McDonald & Collins, 2000; McDaniel & Gee, 1993). It is
difficult to accurately estimate the extent of abuse in homes and institutions across the country. The most current national estimates for Canada
come from the 1999 General Social Survey (Dauvergne, 2003). According to these figures, approximately 1% of seniors experience violence, 7% experience emotional abuse, and 1% experience financial
abuse. This data however, underestimates the incidence of abuse because it did not include Canadians living in retirement homes or other
institutions, and also, because the data was collected by telephone survey (Dauvergne, 2003). It is impossible to predict whether the aging of
the population will lead to an increase in elder abuse.

Although elder abuse is an acknowledged social issue, there has been
very little attention paid to the role of faith leaders and faith communities in identifying and responding to elder abuse (Podnieks, 2003), nor
has this been a research focus. A search on Medline, CINAHL, and Academic Search Elite revealed no pertinent studies of elder abuse and religion, religious communities or religious leaders, or elder abuse and
faith leaders, or faith communities. A study of suicide rates among the
elderly which compares Catholic and Orthodox countries to non-Catho-
lic and non-Orthodox countries hints at the connection. The authors argue that although we might expect Catholic and Orthodox countries to
have *lower* elder suicide rates this was not the case. The findings suggest
to the authors the possibility of an undercurrent of "inadvertent neglect"
(Pritchard and Baldwin, 2000).

A study of the shelter needs of Ontario women conducted in 1998
suggest that faith leaders could indeed be an important group in an overall strategy to identify and intervene in cases of elder abuse. The study,

conducted by the Ontario based Older Women's Network interviewed 106 women speaking 15 different languages in 5 communities across Ontario about their experience with elder abuse. The women were asked where they would turn for help. A surprisingly high number indicated that they would seek support from their religious community. Of the respondents under the age of 76 years, 33% said they would turn to their place of worship for help. Fifty-two percent of those over the age of 76 indicated place of worship as a source of support (Kapel Ramji Consulting Group, 1998).

We suggest that faith leaders could have a key role in the intervention and prevention of abuse. Older Canadians may to look to their faith leader for help in the case of abuse, and a case can be made that religious leaders are indeed obliged to support their followers who suffer abuse. Clergy however, have remained almost universally silent on the topic of elder abuse. A national American study that compared 14 different occupational groups who work with seniors, ranked clergy as among the least effective in addressing elder abuse issues (Blakely & Dolan, 1991). The authors also assert that clergy are among the least likely to refer abuse and/or neglect cases to outside agencies (Blakely & Dolan, 1991). Nason-Clark (1997) and Pagelow and Johnson (1988) caution that clergy may provide inappropriate advice that puts victims of violence at continued risk. According to Nason-Clark (1977), abused Christian women face the unique problem of finding support that recognizes both the experience of violence and their commitment to faith. Religious women who seek help from a religious leader are too often disappointed. Nason-Clark (1977) states, "The response of pastors has been ineffectual at best, while sometimes clergy are guilty of sending a woman back home to a continued cycle of violence" (p 19).

The present study and its companion, published in this volume, were designed to explore faith leaders' experiences of and responses to elder abuse. The first study is based on interviews with faith leaders and parish nurses conducted in Metropolitan Toronto. This study is a survey of faith leaders across the province of Ontario. Although the research strategies are different, the goals have been similar. In both cases we wanted to gain an understanding of faith leaders' perceptions of elder abuse, to ask how faith leaders respond to elder abuse in their communities, to determine what barriers they experience, and to find out what resources faith leaders would find helpful in meeting the needs of their congregants regarding elder abuse (Podnieks, 2003). We use the term "faith leader" to include priest, rabbi, imam, pastor, and other advisors recognized by a faith group. The term may not apply to religious groups where leadership rotates. We assume that religious institutions and their leaders could offer enormous support to abused parishioners if clergy had the information and the skills to address the needs of this large and generally unacknowledged population. In both cases the work is exploratory. Findings from these studies could serve as a modest first step to developing an inclusive and collaborative response to the problem of elder abuse as it relates to faith communities.

THE STUDY

This study was conducted in collaboration with the Ontario Women's Network and the Women's Interfaith Dialogue/The League for Human Rights B'Nai Brith Canada. The advisory committee included members of a wide cross section of community groups and educational institutions including; the University of Toronto's Faculty of Social Work, Ryerson University, Faculty of Community Services, the Ontario Network for the Prevention of Elder Abuse, and representatives from numerous multicultural faith groups, elder abuse networks and senior's organizations. The study was generously funded by Health Canada. The study received approval from the Ethics Review Committees of the University of Toronto and Ryerson University.

The Centre for Applied Social Research (CASR), Faculty of Social Work, University of Toronto was contracted to collect the data. The study design called for a purposive sample of faith leaders in Ontario, Canada. Lists of faith leaders were compiled with the assistance of the multidisciplinary community advisory board and community contacts with faith communities willing to participate in the study. The study team compiled lists of faith organizations from directories (i.e., Yearbook of Religious Organizations, community directories, and Internet searches). The CASR staff in collaboration with the principal investigators and the advisory committee developed the survey instruments (see Appendix).

Interviewers were hired and trained for this study by CASR staff. The interview team members had social work training, as well as experience working directly with multi-cultural populations. The study was conducted in late 1999 and early 2000. It was very difficult to secure time with faith leaders to respond to a questionnaire on the topic of elder abuse. The refusal rate was approximately 40% and each contact required 6 to 10 phone calls before the face to face or telephone meeting could be scheduled. In the end, a total of 49 surveys were completed with faith leaders across the province of Ontario. Twenty-six respondents lived in the City of Toronto, 4 in the Greater Toronto Area, 5 in Southwestern Ontario, 5 in Central Ontario, 6 in Eastern Ontario, and 3 lived in Northern Ontario. Clearly, this sample size is less than ideal, despite the wide geographical representation. As was evident in the companion study faith leaders are extremely busy and have little discretionary time. We do not know whether a reluctance to discuss the issue of elder abuse influenced the low commitment rate.

Faith leaders living in Metropolitan Toronto were interviewed face to face using the questionnaire as guide. Those located outside the City of Toronto responded to the questionnaire by telephone. Two respondents completed the questionnaire by mail at their request. The interviews were audio-taped, with the permission of the respondent. The quantitative data was coded and entered into an SPSS data file. Responses to open-ended questions were transcribed for coding and analysis.

Faith leaders who agreed to answer the survey represented a wide range of religious cultural groups, reflective of the cultural and religious diversity of the province. According to the 2001 census, 34.9% of people living in Ontario are Protestant; 34.3% are Roman Catholic, 16% have no religion and the remaining 14.8% were other Christian, Muslim, Jewish, Buddhist, Hindu, or Sikh (Statistics Canada, 2003:18). These figures were not available at the time the study was being conducted, and they reflect a very dynamic picture when compared with previous numbers. Between the 1991 and 2001 census the proportion of Protestants in the province decreased by over 8%, and the proportion of "other" increased by over 6%. Census figures reflect affiliation only and are not representative of actual attendance. For the country as a whole, only 32% of the population aged 15 years and older attend religious services at least once a month (Clark, 2003:3).

In this study, 68% of the faith leaders were Protestant, 14.6% were Roman Catholic, and 17.1% were Jewish. The sample cannot be considered representative of the population in terms of religious affiliation. We do not have accurate figures for attendance although it remains the case that seniors have the highest attendance rates across all age groups. While unsuccessful in contacting a large, representative sample of faith leaders, the researchers were able to survey the opinions of forty-nine faith leaders representing a wide range of faith groups covering a large geographical area. It is hoped that subsequent studies will seek opinions from additional non-Christian groups, and work with representative samples. The following discussion is based on the results of the survey responses of the forty-nine faith leaders. Representative comments recorded from questionnaires are included in the discussion where appropriate.

FINDINGS

The religious communities represented by the faith leaders in this sample ranged from very small (30 members) to very large (6,400 members). While most congregants spoke English, nine respondents reported that seniors in their faith communities prefer to speak Arabic, Cantonese, German, Greek, Ojibway, Anishinabe, and Portuguese. Faith leaders represented congregants from the following ethnic groups: German, Greek, Portuguese, Chinese, Japanese, Korean, and Taiwanese, Caribbean and Aboriginal Peoples.

All faith leaders mentioned that their members included older adults. Participants were asked, "Where are you most likely to have significant personal contact with seniors in the congregation/faith community that you serve?" Typically faith leaders engaged with seniors in the traditional roles of a religious leader. However respondents mentioned other activities such as informal prayer groups, meetings or just calling to chat with a senior. The greatest contact was either at the place of worship or the senior's home or residence. Other significant personal contacts occurred at funeral homes, meetings, workshops and social activities. One half of the faith communities had programs or activities specifically geared to seniors. These included bereavement or support groups and prayer groups. All respondents said seniors participated in activities open to the general congregation/faith community. Barriers to involvement identified by the faith leader included poor physical health, a physical disability, transportation difficulties, inclement weather, and language barriers.

When asked, "What are you least comfortable asking members of your congregation/faith community about?" one-third (n = 15) said that there were no subjects that fell into this category. Less than one-third (n = 14) were uncomfortable asking about financial issues, including subjects about wills or financial matters after death. Five participants mentioned being uncomfortable talking about sexual issues and preferences; 6 (13%) mentioned family conflicts; 3 commented about issues related to the members' personal life, such as alcohol or drug abuse and 2 mentioned elder abuse situations. Two participants made comments about issues related to the congregation/faith community such as congregational turmoil, and fundraising.

FAITH LEADERS
KNOWLEDGE OF AND EXPERIENCE
WITH ELDER ABUSE

Generally, faith leaders were familiar with the concept of elder abuse and were able to describe parameters including neglect. About one-half of the faith leaders mentioned that their training involved courses or sessions on issues pertaining to older people or gerontology. Specific comments describing the nature of elder abuse included the following: "The senior is put into a degrading environment where they are not able to care for themselves, over-medication or inappropriate use of drugs." Some thought of abuse as taking advantage of an older adult: "Abusing an older person, taking advantage of persons because of age, to manipulate, or cajole a person who is lonely or incapacitated out of their money and resources." A few respondents mentioned that elder abuse could be subtle: "Abuse takes a lot of forms–neglect, sexual, physical, emotional, taking advantage of an elder in a number of different ways, not always clear though." Interestingly, one faith leader commented that even clergy could take advantage of elderly members of their communities: "Violation whether physical or psychological, things happening to seniors against their wishes or desires–can even be clergy–sometimes ministers are especially friendly to seniors to gain financially."

To determine the faith leaders' experience with elder abuse in their congregation/faith community, respondents were asked, "In the last year, what types of inappropriate behaviour toward a member of your congregation/faith community do you know of or suspect?" Approximately two-thirds (63%, n = 30) of the faith leaders knew or suspected abuse among the elder members of their community. Table 1 shows the type of abuse respondents had encountered. The most frequently encountered types of elder abuse were psychological abuse, financial abuse, and neglect.

BARRIERS TO ASKING FOR HELP

Faith leaders were asked their opinions about barriers preventing older people in abusive situations from asking for help. In the opinion of faith leaders, abused seniors do not seek help because they are embarrassed, they fear reprisal, or they feel hopeless about the situation, and feel that it would not change even if they complained. Respondents also wondered if older adults might worry that their complaint might not be

TABLE 1. Types of Abuse Known/Suspected by Faith Leaders in the Last Year Within Congregation

Type of Abuse	Number Suspecting Abuse	Number with Knowledge of Abuse
Psychological Abuse–threat of injury, unreasonable confinement, punishment, or verbal intimidation/humiliation, resulting in mental anguish (e.g., anxiety or depression).	2	14
Financial Exploitation–an improper course of conduct with or without informed consent of the older adult that results in monetary, personal, or other gain for the perpetrator, or monetary, personal, or other loss for the older adult (e.g., theft of personal property, unauthorized bank withdrawals).	2	13
Neglect–the deprivation by a caretaker (family/professionals) of goods or services, which are necessary to maintain physical or mental health (e.g., abandonment or denial of food, over/under medication, or other health related services).	5	13
Violation of Rights–denying elderly people the right to make personal decisions or the right to privacy	-	8
Physical Abuse–non-accidental use of physical force, resulting in injury (e.g., slapped, bruised, cut, burned, physically restrained).	0	5
Sexual Abuse–sexual contact that results from threats, force, or against the elderly persons will (e.g., assault, rape, sexual harassment).	-	1

taken in confidence. Faith leaders suggested the following as barriers for seniors: a false sense of loyalty, embarrassment, love for the abuser, fear of intervention, unwillingness to bother the pastor, and privacy ("the older generation is private"). One faith leader thought the main barrier was shame, ("don't air your linen in public"). Another thought that older adults feared retaliation by family members or caregivers. Another faith leader from a community outside of Toronto said, "If the family member is the abuser, the family member will be known to the priest as it is a small community, therefore, the senior feels disloyal and guilty at disclosure."

FAITH LEADERS' RESPONSES TO ELDER ABUSE

Faith leaders reported a high awareness of elder abuse in their communities. Over 90% *(n = 47)*, of the faith leaders reported they would take some action if they suspected abuse or if abuse was disclosed to them. Table 2 shows their responses to suspected or reported cases of abuse.

The faith leaders in this sample said their first reaction to a situation of suspected abuse would be to investigate the situation. As one explained, I would clarify to find out what's going on. Another said, "I would explore with client what happened and monitor the situation; make calls to other caregivers to explore further." A Catholic priest mentioned that he is required to report this kind of information to his bishop. His response to learning of an abuse situation would be to provide emotional and spiritual support to seek help from community resources, and finally to support the individual to report the situation to authorities.

Many of the participants said their actions depended on the situation. One respondent mentioned that the disclosed abuse is not always true: "I had an experience where an abuse wasn't really true, after investigating further, discussing with family members involved, they were not the perpetrators." When abuse is disclosed during confession, Roman Catholic priests are placed in a quandary, as they cannot act on the disclosure without the permission of the elder.

Typically, faith leaders seek help in addressing cases of abuse in their communities. Over 70% (n = 32) of the respondents said they would enlist other members of the congregation/faith community to assist in pro-

TABLE 2. Faith Leaders Response to Suspected or Disclosed Elder Abuse

Response to Abuse	If you come across a situation where you suspect possible elder abuse what do you generally do? **Number replying yes**	When an older member of your congregation/faith community discloses abuse to you, what is generally the action you take? **Number replying yes**
Investigate further	88% (n = 42)	67% (n = 32)
Provide support/ counselling	52% (n = 23)	56% (n = 27)
Monitor the situation	31% (n = 15)	33% (n = 16)
Refer to a medical professional/social service agency, etc.	50% (n = 24)	31% (n = 15)
Intervene, take action, call police	21% (n = 10)	17% (n = 8)

viding help to an older member who has experienced abuse. As Table 2 shows, half of the faith leaders would refer the situation to an outside person or agency. Faith leaders were asked what outside agencies they have called upon in the past in cases of elder abuse. These responses are shown in Table 3. Half of the respondents reported that they would call service agencies that provide help to seniors.

Respondents in this study were asked about how their religious beliefs, practices or role affect their response to elder abuse. Many mentioned the principle of honouring or caring for elders. For example, a rabbi said, "Judaism focuses on honouring elders, taking care of those who need support." A Christian minister made a similar point by stating, "Scripture teaches us to emphasize caring for the elderly. We have a heightened sense of responsibility for elders. We should think of ourselves as shepherds to a flock, imitate Jesus Christ in caring for others needs."

INFORMATION, TRAINING, AND RESOURCES

Many respondents reported the need for more information and education. As one faith leader said, "There needs to be more information regarding elder abuse to bring it out of the closet. More education is needed." Another respondent suggested an active publicity campaign by seniors' organizations. Most agreed that there is not enough public awareness concerning the issue of elder abuse. In some cases, there had been concerted effort within the faith community to reach seniors–although this did not include a specific focus on abuse. For example, in the Diocese of Toronto, the Age in Action program targets the elderly,

TABLE 3. Outside Agencies or People Called Upon in Cases of Elder Abuse

What outside agencies or people have you called upon to help a member of your congregation/faith community that is experiencing elder abuse?	Number Responding Yes
Service agency	24
Other health professional	8
Police (law enforcement)	7
Physician	6
Lawyer	4
None	5

and involves a concerted effort for a senior ministry. One respondent mentioned that faith leaders are always concerned about "the silent senior–the victim." Faith leaders also consult with one another regarding problematic situations.

The last series of questions related to resources and supports that the faith leaders think would be helpful for themselves or for older members of the community experiencing abuse or family members of a senior who experienced abuse. Table 4 illustrates the type of educational materials about elder abuse faith leaders felt would be useful. Many of the faith leaders mentioned that the materials available must be easy to read, large print, short, translated into the seniors' language and accessible to seniors and their families. As one respondent commented,

TABLE 4. Educational Needs Regarding Elder Abuse

Educational materials that you feel would be helpful:	An older member of your congregation/ faith community who is experiencing abuse?	Family member of a senior who is experiencing abuse in your congregation/ faith community?	You as a faith leader?
	% Mentioned (n)	% Mentioned (n)	% Mentioned (n)
Pamphlets/brochures	75% (n = 36)	73% (n = 35)	42% (n = 20)
Books	21% (n = 10)	29% (n = 14)	25% (n = 12)
Newspapers or magazine articles	17% (n = 8)	23% (n = 11)	10% (n = 5)
Articles in church/ community newsletters	25% (n = 12)	27% (n = 13)	10% (n = 5)
T.V. or radio programs, information commercials	21% (n = 10)	33% (n = 16)	6% (n = 3)
Videos	35% (n = 17)	31% (n = 15)	17% (n = 8)
Audio tape cassettes	17% (n = 8)	17% (n = 8)	4% (n = 2)
Multimedia kits	8% (n = 4)	10% (n = 5)	4% (n = 2)
Database of community services	29% (n = 14)	38% (n = 18)	31% (n = 15)
Internet sites	13% (n = 6)	23% (n = 11)	4% (n = 2)
Hotlines	4% (n = 2)	-	-
Speakers, Support Groups, Workshops, Conferences	15% (n = 7)	13% (n = 6)	3% (n = 3)
List of contact numbers, posters	8% (n = 4)	10% (n = 5)	2% (n = 1)
Other, please specify:	6% (n = 3)	4% (n = 2)	2% (n = 1)

"Something with phone-numbers-helpline, something easy to read and short, to know what's out there, to know that they have to remove themselves from an abusive situation."

A few respondents mentioned that information about the signs of abuse would be useful, to help them know what to look for. They also wanted suggestions about how to approach family members when abuse is suspected. One wanted "suggestions of how to approach the family member, how to see the signs, let them talk about it." Another mentioned the importance of "clarifying what is appropriate and inappropriate, knowing their rights in order to respond, assuring that the elderly person's concerns are not violated." In addition, faith leaders wanted information about resources available in the community and case studies of how to approach both abusers and abused in abusive situations. For some, the information gap was large. One faith leader said he wanted to know, "Where to turn? What are the resources? What are the laws? Are there support groups? Where does one report such thing?" Another stated his needs simply: "What to do if one suspects or knows about it? (see Table 5).

The majority (94%, n = 44), felt that educational materials for the congregation or faith community at large should be made available. Respondents mentioned a range of specific types of educational materials including pamphlets, articles and posters, videos, or television programs. A variety of suggestions were elicited from the participants as to what they felt was the best way to disseminate these materials. The faith leaders suggested mailing information about elder abuse to seniors, having posters and printed material in places seniors frequent, including inserts in church bulletins or newsletters, seminars, and information about elder abuse disseminated through the media. Three-quarters of

TABLE 5. Accessibility Considerations

What considerations would have to be taken into account in providing information about elder abuse to ensure that the materials are accessible in your congregation/faith community?	% YES (n)
Large print booklets, accessible formats for audio disabilities	75% (n = 36)
Accessible places (e.g., banks, libraries, senior centres, dentist/doctors' offices, grocery store bulletin board, hairdressers, etc.)	50% (n = 24)
Cultural/Religious sensitivity	42% (n = 20)
Language	38% (n = 18)
Simple and short formats	12% (n = 6)

the faith leaders felt large print booklets videos or audiotapes should be made available to ensure accessible elder abuse information. One-half of the respondents mentioned that the material should be accessible in places seniors frequent.

ADVOCACY

The last question asked was: "What do you think would be helpful in increasing the existence and efficacy of advocacy for the issue of elder abuse in your congregation/faith community?" The most frequently mentioned strategy was education. An example of a respondent's view about the importance of education was: "Education to ensure that it's not happening, advocate for the rights of seniors. The way the outside world looks at seniors is abhorrent, seniors are a world resource that should never be discarded." One faith leader conveyed the need for a proactive approach in the following way: "What we need in the broad sense is proactive work in the community, to go to people within the congregation to rally around the abused person." Other respondents articulated the need for more information about elder abuse: "Awareness through information, television ads." "We need information about what consists elder abuse. This is not right. What's inappropriate, how does one respond?" One (but only one) respondent mentioned the need to speak to the faith community about abuse, "from the pulpit, connected to the gospels in order to raise the consciousness level of the parish." Clearly, this sample of faith leaders do not see their role as a leadership one in breaking the silence around issues of elder abuse.

Faith communities and faith leaders are important pieces of the puzzle in seeking solutions to the hidden problem of elder abuse. Faith leaders are uniquely positioned to engender the trust of their congregants whether they live in private homes or institutions. This study, based on a purposive sample of faith leaders in Ontario, representing a range of denominations spread across the province was designed to determine the perceptions of faith and religious leaders of elder abuse, the actions taken by them in response to suspected or disclosed situations of elder abuse and their knowledge and understanding of resources and services available for elder abuse intervention.

The results of the study revealed a high awareness of abuse in their communities. Two-thirds of the clergy knew of or suspected elder mistreatment among their parishioners. The most frequently mentioned were psychological and financial abuse and neglect. Least frequently mentioned were physical and sexual abuses. Typical responses to elder abuse included further investigation, counselling and referral. These are interesting responses given the general expression of need for education and information. Faith leaders identified lack of education about elder mistreatment, lack of knowledge and/or skill in intervention techniques, and confidentiality issues as barriers to responding effectively to the abuse of elders.

A publication by the National Center of Elder Abuse (NCEA, 1995), suggests that faith communities are particularly significant resources for older members of minority groups. NCEA (1995), argues that religious faith provides a framework for understanding the external world, and a way in which people can be helped to deal with pain, stress, and injustice. In addition, the guide talks about the fact that, in most cultures, the Church serves not only a religious but also a social function. It is a vehicle for matching resources with those in need through internal formal structures, such as announcements during worship, fellowship groups and Sunday school classes, and through the informal networking of congregation members. It is through this combination of religious and social outreach that faith leaders might be expected to have a significant impact regarding the issue of elder abuse. If they were well informed, they could in turn influence senior congregants and their family members to be proactive in preventing elder abuse.

CONCLUSIONS

During the past two decades, the issue of the mistreatment of older persons has become more widely recognized. Faith communities have not general been seen as resources for addressing problems of elder abuse. The findings of this study suggest that faith leaders are keenly aware of abuse situations in their communities and would welcome strategies for supporting community members who suffer abuse. Faith leaders confirm that elder abuse awareness and education are needed for themselves and their communities, and affirm the need for outreach initiatives and educational materials that are culturally relevant. Despite the shortcomings of the study, the findings provide insight into ways of addressing elder abuse in faith communities. The paper reinforces the importance of recognizing the extent of abuse in faith communities and the potential for faith leaders to be key partners in identifying and supporting those who are experiencing abuse, and in the long run, implementing strategies for change.

REFERENCES

Clark, W. (2003). Pockets of Belief: Religious Attendance Patterns In Canada. *Canadian Social Trends, Spring (68)*, 2-5.

Dauvergne, M. (2003). Family Violence Against Seniors. *Canadian Social Trends, Spring (68)*, 10-14.

Dunlop, B., Rothman, M., Condon, K., Hebert, K., & Martinez, I. (2000). Elder abuse: Risk factors and use of case data to improve policy and practice. *Journal of Elder Abuse and Neglect.* 12 (3/4), 95.

Kapel Ramji Consulting Group. (1998). Study of shelter needs of abused older women. *Executive Summary.* Toronto, ON: Older Women's Network.

McDaniel, S.A., & Gee, E.M. (1993). Social policies regarding caregiving to elders: Canadian contradictions. *Journal of Aging & Social Policy.* 5 (1-2), 57-72.

McDonald, L., & Collins, A. (2000). *Abuse and Neglect of Older Adults: A Discussion Paper.* Ottawa: Health Canada. The National Clearinghouse on Family Violence, 18-19.

Nason-Clark, N. (1997). *The Battered Wife: How Christians Confront Family Violence.* Louisville: Westminster John Knorr Press.

National Centre on Elder Abuse. (1995). *To Reach Beyond Our Grasp: A Community Outreach Guide for Professionals in the Field of Elder Abuse Prevention.* Washington, D.C.

Pagelow, M.D. (1988). Abuse of the elderly in the home. *Abuse and Religion: When Praying Isn't Enough.* (pp. 29-37) A.L. Horton, & J.A. Williamson, (Eds.) Massachusetts: DC. Heath and Company.

Pagelow, M.D., & Johnson, P. (1988). Abuse in the American family: The role of religion. *Abuse and Religion.*(pp. 1-11) A.L. Horton, & J.A. Williamson, (Eds.) Massachusetts: D.C. Heath & Company.

Pagelow, M.D., & Johnson, P. (1988). Abuse in the American Family: The Role of religion. *In Abuse and Religion: When Praying Isn't Enough.* (pp. 1-11) A.L. Horton & J.A. Williamson, (Eds.) Massachusetts: D. C. Heath and Company.

Podnieks, E., Elder Abuse in Faith Communities. Paper presented at the 56th annual scientific meeting of the Gerontological Society of America, San Diego, CA, USA, November 21-25.

Pottie Bunge, V. (2000). Abuse of older adults by other family members. *Family Violence in Canada: A Statistical Profile, 2000.* V. Pottie Bunge, & D. Locke (Eds.). Statistics Canada Catalogue No. 85-224.

Pritchard, C., and D. Baldwin (2000). Effects Of Age And Gender On Elderly Suicide Rates In Catholic And Orthodox Countries: An Inadvertent Neglect? *International Journal of Geriatric Psychiatry.* 15(10): 904-910.

Statistics Canada. (2003). Religions in Canada. Catalogue no. 96F0030XIE2001015. Ottawa: Minister of Industry.

APPENDIX

A. Background Information on the Faith/Religious Congregation/Faith Community. First, I would like to ask you about the congregation/faith community in which you serve.

A1.   What is the faith/religious community that you serve? *(e.g., Catholic, Protestant, Muslim, Sikh, Jewish, etc.)*

A2.   What is the approximate size of your congregation/faith community? _____*number of members*

A3.   Approximately what proportion of your congregation/faith community are seniors (65 years+)? _____%

A4.   What is the main ethnic group to which the majority of the seniors belong in your congregation/faith community?

A5.   What are the main languages the seniors prefer to speak?

A6.   Are there services/programs/activities available through the *(church, mosque, synagogue)* that are specifically geared to seniors?

   0 No

   1 Yes

   A6a. If yes, what are they?

A7.   Are there services/programs/activities open to the general congregation/faith community but are attended by seniors?

   0 No

   1 Yes

   A7a. If yes, what are they?

A8.   Are there any reasons why seniors are not involved in support services/programs in the congregation/faith community you serve? *(e.g., language barriers, no older people in the community, etc.)*

B. Background Information on the Faith/Religious Leader.
Now I would like to ask you about your role as a faith/religious leader.

B1.   What is the proper or full title of your position?

B2.   How many years have you been a faith/religious leader in this congregation/faith community?

   1. less than 5 years

2. 5-10 years

3. 11-20 years

4. 21-29 years

5. 30 + years

B3.   Is your position. . .

1. full time? OR
2. part-time?

B4.   What was your preparation for your position?

B4a. Where?

B4b. How many years? _____(*enter the number of years*)

B4c. Did any of your training involve courses or session on issues of older people or gerontology?

0 No
1 Yes

B4d. If yes, please describe.

B5.   How many years have you been a faith/religious leader?

1. less than 5 years

2. 5-10 years

3. 11-20 years

4. 21-29 years

5. 30 + years

B6.   Where are you most likely to have significant personal contact with seniors in the congregation/faith community that you serve? *(Do not read list but check all that apply: Use the list as probes: Record any comments made verbatim)*

	No	Yes
a. At place of worship	0	1
b. In their own homes	0	1
c. In the homes of their children/extended family	0	1
d. In seniors centers	0	1
e. In nursing homes or other long-term care facilities	0	1
f. In hospital	0	1
g. Other, please specify:	0	1

APPENDIX (continued)

B7. Please list the major activities in which you engage with the seniors of your congregation/faith community? *(Do not read list but check all that apply: Use the list as probes: Record any comments made verbatim)*

	No	Yes
a. Spiritual advisor	0	1
b. Counseling	0	1
c. Ministering to the sick	0	1
d. Concrete help *(e.g,. helping with activities of daily living)*	0	1
e. Recreational/social activities	0	1
f. Other, please specify:	0	1

B8. Amongst all of your duties as a faith/religious leader, what percentage of your time and effort do you think is spent on these activities with seniors per week? _____%

B9. What are you least comfortable asking members of your congregation/faith community about?

C. Faith/Religious Leaders Perceptions and Knowledge about Elder abuse.

Now I would like to move on to your perceptions of elder abuse. I am going to read you two vignettes and then ask you some questions after each vignette.

Vignette 1

While visiting an elderly woman in his congregation in the hospital, the women told the faith leader that she rang repeatedly for the nurse to help her up to the bathroom. Finally arriving an hour later, the nurse told her that the staff was too busy, and said the elder women would have to wait.

C1a. Do you think this is an abusive situation?
   0 No
   1 Yes

C1b. If yes, as a faith leader would you take any action?
   0 No
   1 Yes

C1c. If yes, what action?

C1d. If no, please explain.

Vignette 2

An elderly member of a religious organization, who is confined to his apartment with a respiratory infection, tells his faith leader that a neighbor offered to do the shopping for him. Then the neighbor offered to go to the bank for him. The bank manager was called to O.K. the neighbor cashing a check. The elderly man was surprised to find out that $600 was missing from his account and the bank manager confirmed that the neighbor had withdrawn that money.

C2a. Do you think this is an abusive situation?
0 No
1 Yes

C2b. If yes, as a faith leader would you take any action?
0 No
1 Yes

C2c. If yes, what action?

C2d. If no, please explain.

C3. What does the term elder abuse mean to you?

C4. In the last year, what types of inappropriate behavior toward a member of your congregation/faith community do you know of or suspect of. *(Do not read list but check all that apply: Use the list as probes: Record verbatim any comments made–Probe know of, or suspect)*

	None	Suspect	Know of abuse
a. Physical abuse–non-accidental use of physical force, resulting in injury (e.g., slapped, bruised, cut, burned, physically restrained)	0	1	2
b. Psychological abuse–threat of injury, unreasonable confinement, punishment, or verbal intimidation/humiliation, resulting in mental anguish (e.g., anxiety or depression).	0	1	2
c. Sexual abuse–sexual contact that results from threats, force, or against the elderly persons will (e.g., assault, rape, sexual harassment).	0	1	2

APPENDIX (continued)

d. Financial exploitation–an improper course of conduct with or without informed consent of the older adult that results in monetary, personal, or other gain for the perpetrator, or monetary, personal, or other loss for the older adult (e.g., theft of personal property, unauthorized bank withdrawals).	0	1	2
e. Neglect–the deprivation by a caretaker (family/professionals) of goods or services, which are necessary to maintain physical of mental health (e.g., abandonment or denial of food, over/ under medication, or other health related services)	0	1	2
f. Violation of Rights–denying elderly people the right to make personal decisions or the right to privacy	0	1	2
g. Other, please specify:	0	1	2

C5. Sometimes people are afraid to ask for help with situations of abuse. What are some of the barriers that you think might prevent older people from asking you as the faith/religious leader for help in the congregation/faith community that you serve?

C6. Do you think that members of your congregation/faith community are aware of or have some knowledge about elder abuse?
   0 No
   1 Yes
   C6a. Please describe.

D. Faith/Religious Leaders Responses to Elder abuse
In this section, I would like to ask you some questions about responses to elder abuse.

D1. If you come across a situation where you suspect possible elder abuse what do you generally do? *(Do not read list but check all that apply: Use the list as probes: Record verbatim, any comments made).*

	No	Yes
a. Provide support/counseling	0	1
b. Monitor the situation	0	1
c. Investigate further	0	1
d. Refer to a medical professional/social service agency, etc.	0	1
e. Other, please specify:	0	1

   D1a. Please explain:

D2. When an older member of your congregation/faith community discloses abuse to you, what is generally the action you take? *(Do*

**not read list but check all that apply: Use the list as probes:
Record verbatim any comments made)**

	No	Yes
a. Provide support/counseling	0	1
b. Monitor the situation	0	1
c. Investigate further	0	1
d. Refer to a medical professional/social service agency, etc.	0	1
e. Other, please specify:	0	1

D2a. Please explain:

D3. Do you enlist other members of the congregation/faith community to assist you in providing help to an older member who has experienced abuse?

0 No
1 Yes

D3a. Please explain:

D4. What outside agencies or people have you called upon to help a member of your congregation/faith community that is experiencing elder abuse? *(Do not read list but check all that apply: Use the list as probes: Record verbatim, any comments made)*

	No	Yes
a. None	0	1
b. Physician	0	1
c. Other health professional, please specify:	0	1
d. Lawyer	0	1
e. Police (law enforcement)	0	1
f. Service agency, please specify:	0	1
g. Other, please specify:	0	1

D5. In what way do your religious beliefs, practices or your role as a faith/religious leader, affects your responses to elder abuse in your congregation/faith community? *(e.g., confessional or confidential*

APPENDIX (continued)

nature of the disclosure, sanctity of maintaining the family, role of women, etc.)

D6. From your experience, where do you think an abused senior might go for help if they do not turn to your *(church, mosque, synagogue)*? *(Do not read list but check all that apply: Use the list as probes: Record any comments made verbatim)*

	No	Yes
a. Family Members	0	1
b. Physician	0	1
c. Other health professional, please specify:	0	1
d. Lawyer	0	1
e. Police (law enforcement)	0	1
f. Community center	0	1
g. Service agency, please specify:	0	1
h. Other, please specify:	0	1

D7. Is there any other information regarding you and your congregation/faith community response to elder abuse that you think would be useful?

E. Resources

The next section deals with resource and supports that you or members of your congregation/faith community would find helpful.

Traditionally there are three areas that are perceived as being helpful to an abused senior. I am going to ask you about each area individually.

E1. The first area is educational material.

What educational materials would you feel as being helpful for <u>an older member of your congregation/faith community</u> who is experiencing abuse? *(Do not read list but check all that apply: Use the list as probes: Record verbatim, any comments made)*

	No	Yes
a. Pamphlets/brochures	0	1
b. Books	0	1
c. Newspaper or magazine articles	0	1
d. Articles in church/community newsletters	0	1

	No	Yes
e. T.V. or radio programs, information commercials	0	1
f. Videos	0	1
g. Audio tape cassettes	0	1
h. Multimedia kits	0	1
i. Database of community services	0	1
j. Internet sites	0	1
k. Other, please specify:	0	1

E2. What do you think would be helpful in way of educational materials <u>family members</u> of a senior who is experiencing abuse in your congregation/faith community. **Use the list as probes: Record verbatim, any comments made)** *(Do not read list but check all that apply):*

	No	Yes
a. Pamphlets/brochures	0	1
b. Books	0	1
c. Newspaper or magazine articles	0	1
d. Articles in church/community newsletters	0	1
e. T.V. or radio programs, information commercials	0	1
f. Videos	0	1
·g. Audio tape cassettes	0	1
h. Multimedia kits	0	1
i. Database of community services	0	1
j. Internet sites	0	1
k. Other, please specify:	0	1

E3. What educational materials or information about elder abuse would be helpful <u>to you</u> as a faith/religious leader? *(Do not read list but check all that apply: Use the list as probes: Record any comments made verbatim)*

	No	Yes
a. Pamphlets/brochures	0	1
b. Books	0	1
c. Newspaper or magazine articles	0	1
d. Articles in church/community newsletters	0	1
e. T.V. or radio programs, information commercials	0	1

APPENDIX (continued)

f. Videos	0	1
g. Audio tape cassettes	0	1
h. Multimedia kits	0	1
i. Database of community services	0	1
j. Internet sites	0	1
k. Other, please specify:	0	1

E3a. Please explain:

E4. Do you think that educational materials for the congregation/faith community at large should be made available?

0 No
1 Yes

E4a. If yes, what type of educational material?

E5. What do you think would be the best way to disseminate these materials?

E6. What considerations would have to be taken into account in providing information about elder abuse to ensure that the materials are accessible in your congregation/faith community? *(Do not read list but check all that apply: Use the list as probes: Record verbatim, any comments made)*

	No	Yes
a. Language	0	1
b. Cultural sensitivity	0	1
c. Accessible places (e.g. banks, libraries, senior centers, dentist/ doctors' offices, grocery store bulletin board, hairdressers, etc.)	0	1
d. Large print booklets	0	1
e. Other, please specify:	0	1

E6. The next area is persons and service agency resources. When you think about the people or agencies that you have contacted or would like to contact when dealing with this issue, what resources would be most helpful for you to better assist an older people in your congregation/faith community who has experienced abuse?

E7. What person or agency resources do you think would be most helpful to <u>an older member of </u>your congregation/faith community who has experienced abuse?

E8. The last area is advocacy.
Advocacy in this context is the work that the congregation/faith community or faith/religious leader does to stop the existence of elder abuse.
What do you think would be helpful in increasing the existence and efficacy of advocacy for this issue in your congregation/faith community?

F. Socio-Demographic Profile of the Faith Religious Leader

We are now coming to the end of the interview. I am now going to ask a few questions about you.

F1. Are you . . .
1   Male
2   Female

F2. What is your age?
1. 20-29
2. 30-39
3. 40-49
4. 50-59
5. 60-69
6. 70+

F3. What is your present marital status?
1. Single
2. Married
3. Separated/Divorced
4. Widowed

F4. Were you born in Canada?
1 Yes
0 No

F4a. If no, what is your country of birth?

F5. To which ethnic group do you feel you belong?

F6. What language(s) do you usually speak? (Please list)

F7. What size community do you live in?

1 Rural township or rural municipality

2 Village (less than 1,000 people)

3 Small town (1,000 to 2,499 people)

4 Town (2,500 to 9,999 people)

5 Large town/small city (10,000 to 49,999 people)

6 City (50,000 to 99,999 people)

7 Large city (100,000 people or more)

F8. How long have you lived in this community?

_____(Enter the number of years)

Thank you very much for your time. We will make sure to keep you informed as to the progress of the study and sent you a summary of the results.

Older Women, Domestic Violence, and Elder Abuse: A Review of Commonalities, Differences, and Shared Approaches

Bridget Penhale, MSC, CQSW

SUMMARY. Elder abuse and neglect have increasingly become issues of concern. Older women are the majority of older people who experience abuse, yet there have been few attempts to adequately consider this. Consideration of the potential links between domestic violence and elder abuse is appropriate. This article provides an overview of knowledge about elder abuse and neglect and then moves to examine factors from domestic violence. An exploration, through review, of the similarities and differences between these approaches will assist in determining relative strengths and weaknesses. This will then contribute towards greater understanding of the linked phenomena of elder abuse and neglect and assist towards both protection and prevention of abuse. *[Article copies available for a fee from The Haworth Document Delivery Service: 1-800-HAWORTH. E-mail address: <docdelivery@haworthpress.com> Website: <http://www. HaworthPress.com> © 2003 by The Haworth Press, Inc. All rights reserved.]*

Bridget Penhale is Senior Lecturer, Social Work Faculty of Health and Social Care, University of Hull, Hull HU6 7RX, UK (E-mail: B.L.Penhale@hull.ac.uk).

[Haworth co-indexing entry note]: "Older Women, Domestic Violence, and Elder Abuse: A Review of Commonalities, Differences, and Shared Approaches." Penhale, Bridget. Co-published simultaneously in *Journal of Elder Abuse & Neglect* (The Haworth Maltreatment & Trauma Press, an imprint of The Haworth Press, Inc.) Vol. 15, No. 3/4, 2003, pp. 163-183; and: *Elder Abuse: Selected Papers from the Prague World Congress on Family Violence* (ed: Elizabeth Podnieks, Jordan I. Kosberg, and Ariela Lowenstein) The Haworth Maltreatment & Trauma Press, an imprint of The Haworth Press, Inc., 2003, pp. 163-183. Single or multiple copies of this article are available for a fee from The Haworth Document Delivery Service [1-800-HAWORTH, 9:00 a.m. - 5:00 p.m. (EST). E-mail address: docdelivery@haworthpress.com].

KEYWORDS. Elder abuse, gender, domestic violence, review, similarities, differences, implications

INTRODUCTION

In recent years, there has been a steady increase in concern about the abuse and neglect of older people. The major focus has been on abuse of elders by their carers in the domestic setting although increasingly there has been consideration of abuse occurring within institutional settings (Glendenning, 1999).

The issue of elder abuse is not either a new or a recent phenomenon (Stearns, 1986), but it is really only since the end of the 1980s that the problem began to be addressed in the UK and a number of developed countries. In addition, it is still comparatively early in the stages of identification of the problem and the development of positive action to combat elder abuse and neglect within the UK and many countries. It was not until the mid 1990s that there was any real indication on the part of governments to recognize that there was a problem requiring attention. For example, in the UK, this occurred in 1993 (DOH/SSI, 1993). And it was not until the work of Whittaker (1995), and Aitken and Griffin (1996) that any work containing feminist analyses of elder abuse began to appear in the UK.

Although a number of western countries (for example, Australia, Canada, Norway, Sweden, U.S.) have been working in the area of elder abuse for some years, other countries have only recently begun to conduct work on this problem. Additionally, feminist analyses of elder abuse have been generally lacking. As traditionally, viewed, elder abuse has been considered from the perspective of social science frameworks, rather than from feminist approaches and analyses, which consider the difficulties that occur due to inequities in gender and power relations between individuals. This latter type of approach is more commonly found in considerations of domestic violence of younger women. An exploration, through review, of the similarities and differences between traditional social science frameworks and feminist approaches, which rather explore problems resulting from inequalities of power within society, will assist in determining the relative strengths and weaknesses of each type of approach.

WHAT IS KNOWN ABOUT ELDER ABUSE?

English doctors initially identified the phenomena of elder abuse and neglect in the mid 1970s (Baker, 1975; Burston, 1977), but it was not until the mid 1980s that the issue was really picked up on there. However, in the USA the issue was recognized from the mid 1970s and began to be researched from then on. This was largely achieved through use of the sociological frameworks that were developed for other forms of family violence.

In considering elder abuse and neglect, we must be mindful that this is a complex and sensitive area to investigate. There are a number of possible reasons for this, including, for example, the fact that comparative and developmental norms can be very difficult to establish for older people (Bennett, 1990). However, a similar situation was also previously found with both child abuse and domestic violence against younger women by men known to them.

Since the middle of the 1980s, feminist analyses of elder abuse began to appear (Vinton, 1993), although generally, early feminist perspectives seemed to prioritize the role of gender over other factors such as age, culture, or race. This did not help in the appreciation of difference between individuals. As has been suggested elsewhere, following Hanmer and Hearn's (1999) typology, much of the early research in this area was either 'gender absent' or 'gender neutral' (Penhale and Parker, 1999). Gender was therefore not adequately considered. The move to perspectives that are 'gender present,' but not essentialist (emphasizing gender to the exclusion of all other factors) has been more difficult to achieve.

Due to problems with definitions and with the research data, it is not wholly appropriate to draw generalizations from results of surveys in the USA (Cloke, 1983). However, to give some idea of the possible size of the problem, originally, the majority of research results from the U.S., using traditional social science methods of enquiry suggested that between 4-10% of the elderly population were either at risk of, or were experiencing, abuse from their caregivers (Gioglio and Blakemore, 1985; Pillemer and Finkelhor, 1988; U.S. House of Representatives, 1981). Nowadays, most U.S. researchers agree that somewhere in the region of 4-5% of the population of older people are potentially affected by abuse or neglect (Lachs and Pillemer, 1995). There is also agreement that the majority of those affected by abuse are women.

DEFINITIONS

It has been difficult to define elder abuse and neglect adequately and so there are currently no standardised definition in existence. One of the major problems seems to concern what should be either included in, or excluded from, the definition (Penhale, 1993). The sorts of questions involved include consideration of whether abuse should refer solely to matters of physical assault, whether such crimes as muggings against older people constitute abuse (Pritchard, 1992) or whether such concepts as 'violation of rights' should be included within definitions.

More recently, discussions have begun to consider abuse and neglect at three distinct levels: Macro, Mezzo, and Micro (Bennett, Kingston, and Penhale, 1997). Macro abuse refers to issues at a societal level: inadequate pensions, restricted access to health and social care, fuel costs, and institutional abuse. All of these issues are broadly encompassed under the sociological frameworks of the political economy of ageing (Phillipson, 1982) and structured dependency theories (Townsend, 1981). For a wider analysis of the disempowering nature of social policies concerning older people see Walker, 1986; Townsend, 1981; analyses concerning older women can be found in Arber and Ginn, 1991; 1995.

The term mezzo abuse considers behaviors, attitudes, and policies inflicted on older people at the community level (see for example Pritchard, 1992). These would include anti-social behaviors like gang abuse, ageism, and forcing people to live what Phillipson (1992) calls 'marginal lives.'

In more general terms, up until the present, attention has usually been focused on elder abuse and neglect at the micro, individual level. This encompassed conflict in later life between two actors, usually in the domestic setting, whether this is the elder's own home or the home of a relative with whom the elder resides.

In future, it is possible that the definition of abuse may be extended to cover a wider range of ideologies and policies that clearly force older people to live on the periphery of society. It is clear also that rather more attention needs to be paid to matters concerning institutional abuse (Phillipson, 1993), although this has begun to develop in recent years (Glendenning, 1999; Stanley et al., 1999).

Despite the difficulties already mentioned, we have seen the emergence of a number of definitions of elder abuse. Within most definitions, the usual types of abuse included are: physical, psychological, financial, and neglect. To this group have been added sexual abuse, as a category separate from physical abuse, and also, within some definitions, social abuse. The types of behavior covered by each category include:

- Physical abuse: The infliction of physical harm, injury, physical coercion, sexual molestation and physical restraint;
- Psychological abuse: The infliction of mental anguish, verbal and emotional abuse;
- Material abuse: The illegal or improper exploitation and/or use of funds or materials, including property;
- Active neglect: The refusal or failure to undertake a care-giving obligation (including a conscious and intentional attempt to inflict physical or emotional stress on the elder);
- Passive neglect: The refusal or failure to fulfil a caretaking obligation (excluding a conscious and intentional attempt to inflict physical or emotional distress on the elder) (Wolf and Pillemer, 1989).

It is also possible to produce a list of indicators of abuse, although it is difficult to diagnose mistreatment using such indicators alone. To link a bruise to mistreatment, for example, would require much more evidence than just the presence of that injury in isolation. However, the presence of an indicator should alert the individual to the possibility that abuse or neglect may have occurred and act as a prompt for further enquiries to take place.

INCLUSION OF GENDER

Throughout the literature that has developed in the past decade, it is generally understood that males are more likely to abuse than women and that women are more likely to be abused than men within situations of elder abuse (Hightower et al., 1999). This may lead to some inference that categorises men as abusers/perpetrators and women as abused/victim. When consideration is simply of numbers, this appears to be clear, but there is a need for abuse to be understood from a wider perspective. This perspective requires understanding of the societal context in which abuse occurs. It would include, for instance an understanding of the possibility that some women are abusers and for some men to be abused (Pritchard, 2000).

Whilst both men and women are abused, the majority of victims of elder abuse are female, even when this is corrected for by the fact that there are more older women in the population. Although there is still uncertainty regarding the rates of elder abuse either as an overall figure or with regard to the various sub-types, it can be stated with some certainty that abuse within the domestic setting occurs across all ethnic and socio-economic groups and in both urban and rural areas (Steuer & Austin, 1980). It is acknowledged however, that in relation to sexual abuse of elders, the majority of those who experience such abuse are women (Teaster et al., 2000).

Those who abuse may be male, female; partners, adult children, or other relatives. As with other forms of familial violence, the majority of abusers are men. When the probability for abuse is corrected for by the amount of time that the abuser spends with the victim, men are much more likely to be involved in abusive acts, particularly physically violent acts (Finkelhor, 1983).

Many early studies of elder abuse indicated that abusers were more likely to be female, usually relatives (Eastman, 1984). From further analyses of such data, including a distinction between physical abuse and neglect it has been established that men were more likely to be involved in physical violence and women in neglectful acts (Miller & Dodder, 1989; Sengstock, 1991). The former researchers suggested that because categories of neglect (including self neglect) were very high in the studies they reviewed, this to a large extent explained why it had appeared that the majority of abusers were women.

Barnett et al. (1997) reviewed research concerning the characteristics of abusers and abused and found rather contradictory results regarding gender. Adult Protective Service figures reveal most victims are female (68%) (Tatara,1993). In the earlier Boston survey, the majority of victims were male (52%) (Pillemer and Finkelhor, 1988), whilst 65% of respondents were female. The victimisation rate for men at 5.1% was double that for women (2.5%) and yet the elderly population was disproportionately female. It must be remembered, however, that women tend to sustain more serious abuse and injuries than men, which may mean that women are more likely to require treatment for their injuries and may thus be much more likely to come to the attention of authorities.

It may be, for example, that women are more likely to report abuse than men or perhaps, to seek assistance. Also, men are more likely to be physically violent and to commit more serious violence than women. And if much elder abuse is between partners in later life, and the principal form of abuse for male abusers is physical violence towards women, then it may appear that more women are abused than men. Abusive behaviour by women that is likely to be psychological or passively ne-glectful in type may not result in any treatment for the male victim and so this may not come to the attention of professionals. As is found for younger women, sexual abuse in later life appears to be highly gendered: Those who are victims are female; those who abuse are male.

One of the acknowledged risk factors for elder abuse concerns living with others and as men are more likely to live with someone else in old age, this may well increase the risk to older men and possibly make abuse of older men more likely. The work of Kosberg (1998) and Prit-chard (2001) in considering the needs of older men who experience abuse is important to note here. This is consistent with research into the characteristics of abusers: Someone who has lived with victim for a long time. The person is most often a relative, usually adult children, spouses, grandchildren, siblings, then other relatives (Tatara, 1993). Pillemer and Finkelhor (1988) found that abuse was mainly between partners in later life and that abuse by non-family members was quite rare (see also Halicka, 1995; Johns and Hydle, 1995).

Kosberg (1998) suggests that in many situations, the motivation of revenge or 'pay back' for previous abuses of power may be apparent. Within such a model, a woman, or children who experienced abuse from a man at an earlier point in their family's history may see abuse as a form of revenge on the man in later life. Swedish researchers Grafstrom, Norberg, and Wimblad (1992) found some evidence for this type of dynamic in their study of caregivers. However, Jack (1994) sug-gests that female-to-female and female-to-male abuse needs to be situ-ated within the context of exchange relationships within a dysfunction-ing and oppressive society.

Traditionally, elder abuse in domestic settings has been perceived as a problem occurring between a female abuser, often a caregiver, and older parents. However, Aitkin's study reported that older women were more likely to be abused by male sons rather than husbands (Aitken and Griffin, 1996). Women were mostly physically abused; men were psy-chologically abused. It is possible that this could reflect gendered be-haviour. Within the literature on elder abuse that follows a family violence model, are found many references to 'dysfunctional families.' Whittaker (1995) suggests that such a view perpetuates the notion that abuse is symptomatic of a malfunctioning family. In her view, such a situation therefore precludes adequate consideration of gender issues.

The potential effects of gender within abuse are influenced by a num-ber of factors. These include the type of abuse which occurs; the fact that there are more older women within the population and that more

women than men live alone in later life (Arber and Ginn, 1991), yet
there is a higher risk of abuse occurring when people live together
(Wolf, 1993). The different types of abuse that elder abuse consists of
also do not help to clarify the role of gender within such situations.

However, we should not view elder abuse simply in the context of
families and interpersonal relationships. The fluid nature of power and
the continuing prevalence of patriarchal assumptions are also linked to
abuse within the context of health and social care. Social and health care
agencies accountable for 'protective responsibility' may overtly or inadvertently abuse (Stevenson and Parsloe, 1993). Additionally, Jack
(1994) suggests that dependence, power and violation characterize the
nature of relationships and that mutual (albeit unequal) dependency,
powerlessness and violation leads to, and maintains abuse by formal
carers.

There have been relatively few attempts until now to really consider
the role of gender within elder abuse (Aitken and Griffin, 1996; Hightower et al., 1999; Hudson, 1997; Leeder, 1994; Mears, 1995; Whittaker, 1995). In an attempt to consider aspects of gender more appropri-
ately, Whittaker suggests that consideration of differing types of abuse,
for example 'family violence' or 'carer stress' leads to a confounding of
the effects of gender (Whittaker, 1995a). It is proposed that the general
concept of 'elder abuse' should be more closely examined and that more
emphasis should be given to the nature of power within relationships.
To follow feminist analyses somewhat further, it is necessary to examine the oppression of women: women being socially, economically, and
politically controlled by men. This control frequently occurs in male violence against women; one aspect of this is abuse between partners in a
relationship (Whalen, 1996). It is necessary to examine the degree to
which such an analysis is appropriate in relation to elder abuse and perhaps more particularly the abuse of older women. As part of this exploration, it is necessary to consider the similarities and differences that
exist between elder abuse and domestic violence.

SIMILARITIES BETWEEN ELDER ABUSE
AND DOMESTIC VIOLENCE

Elder abuse has been more often compared to issues concerning child
protection than to domestic violence, yet there are notable similarities
between elder abuse and abuse of younger women which should be acknowledged. In any case, as seen above, it is apparent that a significant

proportion of elder abuse is abuse between partners in later life where the predominant dynamic is that of domestic violence which is occurring in later life.

Firstly, in both cases, what is being considered is the abuse of adults. The individuals involved are usually adults who are independent, but linked through familial relationships of emotional (if not blood) ties. Shared living arrangements between the parties are usually due to choice. However, some might argue that particularly in relation to older people, this may be more on grounds of moral obligation than absolute freedom of choice and action.

It is important too, not to infantilise either elders or women who experience abuse, or to reduce their situations to those which are based purely on dependence and an equivalent status to those of children. Older people and younger women who are abused are adults and should be accorded full legal status and rights as citizens. They may require assistance to enable them to make full use of this, but the principles of self-determination, autonomy, and empowerment should remain paramount.

The theoretical frameworks which have been developed to investigate the possible causes of different types of abuse are similar, although this may be largely due to attempts to apply the models proposed for other forms of familial violence to elder abuse. Somewhat uncritical assumptions have been made that the theoretical frameworks and explanations from both psychological and sociological disciplines are both comparable and transferable between and across different forms of abuse.

Such frameworks include such theories as Family dynamics/Transgenerational violence; Exchange theories; Stress theories (either internal or external stress for the family and/or the individuals concerned; or a combination of these) and theories which propose individual psychopathology, usually of the abuser, as being crucial in the genesis of abuse. There are also several theories that look at the dependency and powerlessness of the victim of abuse as being important in terms of the causation of abusive situations. A more rigorous feminist analysis has been applied to both domestic violence and issues of child abuse, but until this point this has not been adequately developed within considerations of elder abuse. Such analyses have considered the gendered nature of power relations and inequalities within the production and maintenance of abusive situations. We are beginning to see the development of these in relation to the abuse of older women (Whittaker, 1995b; Mears, 1997; Hightower et al., 1999).

There would also seem to be strong similarities in the characteristics of those individuals who commit abusive acts. Research has indicated that such people often have alcohol and/or drug misuse problems or histories of psychiatric or personality difficulties and associated relationship problems (Pillemer and Wandolf, 1986). There are also rather more tentative suggestions that those who perpetrate elder abuse are likely, as in other forms of domestic violence, to have been subjected to abuse within the family setting at earlier stages of their lives (Pillemer and Suitor, 1988).

The effects of different forms of abuse on victims also appear to show areas of correspondence (even allowing for individual differences in terms of reactions to abuse). Such effects include attitudes of self-blame and stigma; a lowering of self esteem and reduction in the general coping skills of the person. Other effects of note may be depression, sleep disturbances, a sense of isolation and despair, and an increase in feelings of dependence. These can be seen in victims of virtually all forms of familial violence (although not in every situation) and may well relate to such structural issues as the inequalities of power within relationships, which lead to the development of abusive situations.

Within the differing forms of family violence, difficulties have been encountered in terms of establishing appropriate strategies of intervention. There is a societal stigma surrounding abuse (of all types) and this will in all probability lead to a reluctance on the part of those involved in abusive situations to accept or to seek assistance in their predicament. Victims are not infrequently both intimidated by and fearful of their abusers. Their powerless positions (and the associated perception of this) can make it difficult to empower them sufficiently to leave or change an abusive situation. In addition, within some abusive situations, there are levels of attachment and affection, which the parties concerned do not necessarily wish to alter or risk losing through more formal means of intervention to end the abuse.

As we currently understand domestic violence, the phenomenon that occurs most often is male violence directed towards women and in many situations, their children. As seen earlier, even in addition to those situations which may be considered to be domestic violence in later life, or even ". . . graduated domestic violence . . ." (Biggs et al., 1995, p. 45), the majority of victims of elder abuse are female and the majority of abusers, particularly in situations of physical and sexual abuse, are male.

It is clear that although in some situations domestic violence does not continue into later life (often due to separation or divorce), in others the violent and abusive relationship continues into old age. In some of these situations the violence may actually worsen with age; the effects may in fact be more severe, although this may, on occasion, be due to increased frailty and vulnerability on the part of the victim. If an individual's susceptibility to injury increases with age (due to frailty on their part) then the experience and effects of violence may become more serious.

Abusive situations between partners may begin in later life due to changes in the relationship, which are not expected or planned for. The effects of illness, disability or other related trauma on relationships are not always easy to gauge or to anticipate. A relationship that has always been problematic, if not actually abusive, may deteriorate into abuse if unwanted and unexpected limitations and pressures are suddenly thrust upon a couple.

Deteriorating health, both physical and psychological; thwarted hopes, expectations and plans; a diminution in capacities to function and manage; an increase in vulnerability and dependence may all contribute to the development or continuation of abusive situations within intimate relationships in old age. A lack of understanding and knowledge about the effects of an illness or disability, particularly where this is of a progressive nature, may also be of relevance. The issues surrounding caring, dependency, and abuse are of importance and will require further detailed examination and analysis in coming years. This is likely to be assisted by a view, which encompasses the wider structural factors that can precipitate abuse, such as inequalities of power, inadequate resources, and financial inequalities.

The change in attitudes that has occurred in recent years towards different forms of violence is also pertinent here. It is apparent that both domestic violence and elder abuse are now perceived as appropriate fields of concern; moreover, that these are legitimate areas for concern by the general public. What are undoubtedly areas of great private distress for women are increasingly viewed as appropriate arenas for public concern and action.

A further potentially useful set of comparisons can be drawn in terms of consideration of strategies of intervention. Within the sphere of domestic violence, successful use has been made of self-help groups to provide mutual support for victims. This is now being adapted and the potential utility for elders has been tested out in America (Wolf, 1993). In addition, awareness or consciousness-raising has been an important tool within domestic violence more generally, to assert the right of women to live their lives free from violence or the threat of violence. Campaigns such as that launched in the UK in the early part of 1994 entitled "Zero Tolerance" (Lloyd, 1995) have been very useful in promoting the issues concerning domestic violence and might be adapted to future campaigns concerning older women who are or who have been subject to abuse. The development of screening tools and protocols for referrals concerning elder abuse and later life domestic violence (Ejaz et al., 2001) is also likely to be of assistance in relation to this area.

A link might also be fruitfully made when considering the use of refuges or "safe houses" to offer protection for older women who have experienced abuse (Hightower et al., 1999). The major provider of "Battered Women's Refuges" (as they were originally named) in the UK, Women's Aid, has indicated that they do not discriminate on grounds of age and that their services are equally available for older women who have been subject to abuse. However, it may be unlikely for a number of different but inter-related reasons that an older woman would choose to use such a resource. The development of safe houses for older women who have been victims of abuse might have much to commend it as it is based on a very different set of assumptions than the currently predominant model of institutional care as appropriate for elders who have been abused (Cabness, 1989). Progress in this area has been reported in recent years (Hightower et al., 1999) and looks set to continue.

Specifically, the notion that such accommodation should be provided on a temporary basis, to allow the individual some space and a protective, safe environment in which to properly consider the available options before moving on is preferable to the somewhat paternalistic and disempowering views surrounding much existing institutional care for older people. The differences in attitude and philosophical underpinnings associated with this approach might well make this a more attractive option for older women and is already being developed in America (Breckman & Adelman, 1988; Hudson, 1997; Vinton, 1992).

A further area of comparison surrounds the sphere of legal powers that may be used in connection with domestic violence. Despite a traditional reluctance on the part of the police and legal profession to become involved and intervene in situations of violence against younger women, this situation is now altering. The police in particular have become somewhat more pro-active and the establishment of Domestic Violence Units (or as in some places the more aptly named Family Protection Units) is clearly assisting in this process.

The use of legal sanctions such as injunctions for older people to prevent or alleviate abusive situations is an important corollary to this. And of course, older women who experience violence from their partner could use some of the legislation concerning domestic violence. Recent practice experience suggests that there is an increasing willingness to consider and assist older people to make use of the legal remedies available to them and to advise them accordingly. Older women need to be assisted and empowered to make full use of the law, which might serve to protect them.

The final area of correspondence, which it is necessary to highlight, concerns what might be termed the principles of intervention within the different forms of family violence. For all areas, these generally reflect issues surrounding attempts to redress the imbalances of power that arise and exist within abusive situations. Thus all those working with victims of violence are exhorted to work in partnership and participation with individuals in order to resolve difficulties. As Schaffer indicates, linkage between domestic violence interventions and older women's projects can be a useful development (Schaffer, 1999). The current emphases are firmly stated as being to enable and to empower those individuals who are disadvantaged and disempowered by abusive situations. It is crucial to avoid blaming the victim and creating or perpetuating feelings of guilt and stigma. Within such a framework, there needs to be both adequate provision and protection for individuals who are abused in addition to a context in which the prevention of abuse and violence are actively sought. The overall objective is to empower: To assist and enable individuals to live lives free from abuse, neglect, and exploitation with the promotion of full citizenship rights.

It is apparent, however, that the extent of the comparison between elder abuse and domestic violence in more general terms has yet to be fully tested out in terms of the true nature of the correspondence and the limits to this. Some of the reason for this may rest in the very different origins of the two movements: Elder abuse being largely driven by a professional lobby whilst the domestic violence movement is very much political in origin with a background in feminism. Further examination of an empirical nature concerning the exact nature of the similarities and differences is needed in the future in order to provide some clarity around this area.

DIFFERENCES BETWEEN ELDER ABUSE AND DOMESTIC VIOLENCE

There are a number of differences between elder abuse and domestic violence and these need to be considered. Firstly, there are a number of significant differences in the aetiology of abuse, which can be discerned at the level of the individual. The causes of the abuse may be quite different. Many victims of elder abuse are mentally and/or physically frail and dependent, while abused women, although they may be in a dependent situation, do not necessarily have any disability. It should be acknowledged here that disabled women, both old and young are abused, and additionally that some disabled women may have become disabled as a result of the abuse they have experienced (Fawcett, 2002).

In situations involving domestic violence, the relationships are generally comparatively recent in origin, whereas elder abuse very often involves relationships of many years duration. Abusive situations may arise as a result of very long standing difficulties within a relationship (Fulmer and O'Malley, 1987). The time frames in terms of the relationships between individuals are likely to be very different between situations of elder abuse and those of domestic violence of younger women.

Older people may have more economic and emotional independence than is possible for many younger women. This also includes the right to refuse offers of assistance and intervention by professionals. Older people are generally acknowledged as responsible and independent individuals who can take their own decisions. The economic independence of many elderly people may however make them vulnerable to a type of exploitation and abuse, which is rarely seen in other forms of family violence. It must also be borne in mind, however, that the experience of poverty in later life is predominantly a female experience (Arber and Ginn, 1991) so that older women may not necessarily experience more economic independence than younger women.

There are differences, too in terms of treatment approaches to the two forms of abuse. Within many situations of elder abuse, there is an assumption that it is preferable for the elder to remain living at home, with enough support and assistance and empowerment to enable them to be free of abuse, whilst the goal of much work within situations of domestic violence is to empower the woman sufficiently to enable her to leave the abusive situation. For older women who have experienced domestic violence (regardless of the duration of such abuse, be it short or long term in nature) the aim of intervention may also be empowerment to change the situation, possibly by leaving it.

The initial identification of the two forms of abuse is also of some relevance here, for it was the women's movement of the 1970s, which was instrumental in obtaining recognition of domestic violence as a problem for younger women. By contrast, elder abuse was identified by medical and human services professionals rather than a more 'grassroots' approach. This difference has resulted in different routes in terms of strategies concerning prevention of abuse, protection of and provision for those who are abused. It is possible, too, that the identification and recognition of elder abuse as a social problem may also have been affected.

DIRECTIONS FOR FUTURE RESEARCH

One key area that requires further research is to try and determine the nature of both commonalities and differences between domestic violence and the abuse of older women. This would include a need to explore issues of dependency and vulnerability that women may experience throughout the life-course and how these may alter over time. We need to discover more about why certain people, such as women, people with dementia and other mental and physical health difficulties appear to be at more risk of abuse (Penhale, 1999). Specifically, identification of those factors that seem to render or increase individuals' vulnerability would be helpful in the search to resolve and even prevent abusive situations.

Some useful work is already being undertaken concerning the use of screening tools for abuse of older and younger women (Ejaz et al., 2001). This work could perhaps be extended to other related areas and different assessment formats in relation to responding to abuse. Following consideration of the initial stages of screening and assessment, however, it would also be valuable to consider the extent to which approaches to intervention within abusive situations experienced by women at different stages of the life-course are shared or distinctive and the relative utility of such approaches. Action-research concerning the use of shelters, is one example of such an approach that could be taken here.

It would also appear to be appropriate to examine the links between elder abuse that occurs in domestic settings, with abuse in institutional environments rather more closely. Further investigation of the settings in which abuse may occur would prove useful. Research and subsequent analysis which explores the nature and effects of power within relationships and different situations might find some interesting areas of correspondence between the domestic and the institutional setting. This would add to knowledge and understanding of some important dynamics of abuse.

Furthermore, structural concomitants of abuse, such as the poverty and oppression that many elders experience would appear worthy of further examination. More detailed exploration of aspects relating to gender, power and ethnicity in abusive situations would assist with this (Penhale, 1999). This would be of particular relevance in terms of establishing the extent to which such aspects as these both perpetuate abusive situations and act against their resolution. In addition to this, exploration of the links between the oppression of older people (in particular older women) and that of younger women or disabled people would also be of value in a wider consideration of different aspects of interpersonal violence. This would include those areas that are shared and in common and those that are distinctive to particular forms of violence and abuse. Further understanding of and knowledge about different types of abuse and violence will be useful in the efforts to both resolve and prevent abuse in future.

CONCLUDING COMMENTS

From the above discussion it is clear that elder abuse can be usefully compared to domestic violence, although the exact extent of the correspondence is not yet absolutely clear. A certain amount of caution needs to be employed, however; for example, in order to avoid the development of hasty and inappropriate assumptions and reactions in terms of policy responses.

It is equally apparent, as indicated above, that the extent of the comparison with the wider sphere of domestic violence has not been fully developed to date. That it is appropriate to begin to do so lies in the evident parallels: That of independent adults living together for a number of different but inter-related reasons. In addition, as suggested earlier, much elder abuse would appear to concern abuse between partners in later life (including situations of domestic violence of many years standing). To take such an approach avoids the aforementioned risks of infantilisation; it also allows for an examination of any inter-dependency, which may be required to adequately analyze the dynamics of abusive situations.

In addition, however, concern about elder abuse has arisen over the past ten years or so largely in the context of specialized services and professionals working with older people. It is within this particular context that responses and interventions to alleviate abuse have been developing. Elder abuse is thus viewed as a problem with its own distinctive characteristics, which set it apart from other forms of violence, instead of looking at the evident correspondences between the abuse of older women and violence towards younger women and developing responses in conjunction with these. In this respect, the term elder abuse, by virtue of its gender-neutral status, may disempower older women who are the majority of elders who experience abuse in later life. Links with the feminist movement to end violence against women may serve to empower older women and to promote their rights to full citizenship.

Elder abuse is similar to and yet different from other types of family violence. The nature and extent of the differences suggests that it should still be considered somewhat separately from the totality of family conflict. This should not be taken to promote the isolation of the topic from other forms of abuse and violence, far from it. Moreover, it is also necessary to develop analyses that consider elder abuse as fully as possible in terms of its historical, political, social and cultural contexts.

The spectrum of elder abuse, if viewed as a continuum, encompasses both abuse between partners in later life and child abuse and many variations in between. It also encompasses abuse that occurs within institutions, either due to the regime within the institution, or abuse that occurs directed at an individual in that setting (from a relative, paid carer, or indeed another resident). This form of abuse is indeed different from violence occurring within the domestic setting and is an indication of the extra care that needs to be taken when considering the abuse of older women. Notwithstanding this, however, an analysis which considers the nature and effects of power within relationships and situations might find some areas of correspondence between the domestic and the institutional setting (Jack, 1994), which could then contribute to the development of appropriate strategies for the protection of those who are abused and also the prevention of abuse.

Of importance also within the field of elder abuse are the societal views and attitudes, which are commonly held concerning older people. The discrimination and lowered social status experienced by older people; the routinized devaluation which elders experience from living in an ageist society can exacerbate vulnerability which may already exist due to deterioration in physical and mental health. The risk of abuse may thus be increased for individuals. There is, of course, an additional effect on older women who are subject to further marginalization from a sexist society. As indicated by Walker:

> Ageing society is primarily a female society. It is well known . . . that ageism and sexism combine to produce a socially constructed dependency in older women of which the feminization of poverty is the key feature. (Walker, 1986)

Furthermore, such factors as the wider oppression of older people, and in particular older women, and the lack of resources for them to either avoid or prevent abuse can be seen to interplay with both individual circumstances and any pre-existing psychopathology. This may result in abuse, or may indeed worsen an existing abusive situation.

Such structural concomitants of abuse warrant further attention in terms of the extent to which these aspects both perpetuate abusive situations and militate against their resolution. There is a very real sense in which the wider marginalization of older people within an ageist society is likely to hinder attempts to prevent and alleviate abusive situations.

This paper has considered aspects of elder abuse and domestic violence concerning older women. It is clear that urgent attention should be paid to prevention, protection, where necessary, and strategies of empowerment that are specifically woman-centered. In addition, perhaps more critically, rather more attention must be paid to the nature of power relations in the creation and maintenance of abusive relationships. This is important for all older women who are affected by such violence and, additionally, all those of us whose lives are touched by these experiences.

As is evident at present for older women:

> To be old in the UK is to be marginalized (single jeopardy); to be old and abused is to be marginalized (double jeopardy); to be old and abused and female is to be marginalized (triple jeopardy). (Penhale and Kingston, 1995, p. 237)

To this should be added two further forms of jeopardy: for those women of colour and for those women who are disabled, whether as a result of abuse and violence or not, both of whom experience marginalization and exclusion. Thus there are five potential areas of jeopardy, disadvantage, and disempowerment that older women could face in later life; there may of course be multiple combinations of these. Yet the first three forms of jeopardy may be near universal for women, as they grow older; younger women of course may face up to four possible jeopardies (excluding the experience of the marginalization faced in old age). It is surely time for the feminist movement to assist in developing analyses, and strategies for the provision, protection and empowerment of older women: For all our tomorrows.

REFERENCES

Aitken, L., and Griffin, G. (1996) *Gender and Elder Abuse*, London, Sage.

Arber, S., and Ginn, J. (1991). *Gender and Later Life*, London, Sage.

Arber, S., and Ginn, J. (1995) (Eds.), *Connecting gender and ageing: Sociological approaches to gender relations in later life*, Buckingham, Open University Press.

Baker, A. (1975) Granny Battering, *Modern Geriatrics*. August 5th, (8), 20-24.

Bennett, G. (1990) Action on Elder Abuse in the 1990s: New definitions will help, *Geriatric Medicine*, 20, (4), 53-54.

Bennett, G., Kingston, P., and Penhale, B. (1997) *The Dimensions of Elder Abuse: Perspectives for Practitioners*, Basingstoke, Macmillan.

Biggs, S., Kingston, P.A., and Phillipson, C. (1995) *Elder Abuse in Perspective*, Buckingham, Open University Press.

Breckman, R. S., and Adelman, R. D. (1988) *Strategies for Helping Victims of Elder Mistreatment*. Newbury Park, CA, Sage.

Burston, G. R. (1975) Granny Bashing, *British Medical Journal*, 3 (6): 592.

Cabness, J. (1989) The Emergency Shelter: A model for building the self-esteem of abused elders, *Journal of Elder Abuse & Neglect*, 1, (2), 71-82.

Cloke, C. (1983) *Old Age Abuse in the Domestic Setting–A Review*, Mitcham, Age Concern.

DOH/SSI (Department of Health/Social Services Inspectorate (1993) *No Longer Afraid: The safeguard of older people in domestic settings*, London, HMSO.

Eastman, M. (1984) *Old Age Abuse*, Portsmouth, Age Concern.

Ejaz, F., Bass, D., Anetzberger, G., and Nagpaul, K. (2001) Evaluating the Ohio Elder Abuse and Domestic Violence in Late Life Screening Tools and Referral Protocol *Journal of Elder Abuse & Neglect*, 13, (2), 39-58.

Fawcett, B. (2002) Convergence or Divergence? Responding to the Abuse of Disabled Women, *Journal of Adult Protection*, 4, (3), 24-33.

Finkelhor, D. (1983) Common Features of Family Abuse, in Finkelhor, D., Gelles, R. J., Hotaling, G., and Straus. M. (Eds.), (1983). *The Dark Side of Families: Current Family Violence Research*, Newbury Park, Sage.

Fulmer, T., and O'Malley, T. (1987) *Inadequate care of the elderly: A health care perspective on abuse and neglect*, New York, Springer.

Gioglio, G.R., and Blakemore, P. (1985) *Elder abuse in New Jersey: The knowledge and experience of abuse among older New Jerseyians*. Trenton: New Jersey Division of Youth and Family Services, Bureau of Research and New Jersey Department of Community Affairs, New Jersey Division of Aging.

Glendenning, F. (1999) Elder Abuse and Neglect in Residential Settings: The need for inclusiveness in Elder Abuse research, *Journal of Elder Abuse & Neglect*, 10, (1/2), 1-12.

Grafstrom, M., Norberg, A., and Wimblad, B. (1992) Abuse is in the eye of the beholder. Reports by family members about abuse of demented persons in home care: A total population-based study. *Scandinavian Journal of Social Medicine*, 21, 4, 247-255.

Halicka, M. (1995) Elder Abuse and Neglect in Poland, *Journal of Elder Abuse & Neglect*, 6, (3/4), 157-169.

Hanmer, J., and Hearn, J. (1999) Gender and Welfare Research in Williams, F., Popay, J., and Oakley, A. (Eds.), *Welfare Research: A critical review*, London: UCL Press.

Hightower, J., Smith, M., Ward-Hall, C., and Hightower, H. (1999) Meeting the Needs of Abused Older Women? A British Colombia and Yukon Transition House Survey, *Journal of Elder Abuse & Neglect*, 11, (4), 39-58.

Hudson, M. F. (1997) Elder mistreatment: Its relevance to older women. *Journal of American Medical Women's Association*, 52(3), 142-6, 158.

Jack, R. (1994) Dependence, power, and violation; Gender issues in the abuse of elderly people by formal carers in Eastman, M. (1994) (Ed.), *Old Age Abuse*, London: Chapman Hall.

Johns, S., and Hydle, I, (1995) Norway: Weakness in Welfare, *Journal of Elder Abuse & Neglect*, 6, (3/4), 139-156.

Kosberg, J. (1998) Abuse of Elderly Men, *Journal of Elder Abuse & Neglect*, 9, (3), 69-88.

Lachs, M., and Pillemer, K. (1995) Abuse and Neglect of Elderly Persons, *New England Medical Journal*, 332, (7), 437-443.

Leeder, E. (1994) *Treating Abuse in Families: A Feminist and Community Approach*, New York, Springer Publications.

Lloyd, S. (1995) Social work and Domestic Violence in Kingston, P., and Penhale, B. (1995) (Eds.), *Family Violence and the Caring Professions*. Basingstoke, Macmillan.

Mears, J. (1995) *Triple Jeopardy: Gender and the Abuse of Older People*, University of Western Sydney, Macarthur; Discussion Paper.

Miller, R. B., and Dodder, R. A. (1989) The Abused: Abuser Dyad; Elder Abuse in the State of Florida in Filinson, R. and Ingman, S. R. (Eds.), (1989). *Elder Abuse: Practice and Policy*, New York, Human Sciences Press.

Penhale, B. (1993) The Abuse of Elderly People: Considerations for Practice, *British Journal of Social Work*, 23, 2, 95-112.

Penhale, B. (1999) Researching Elder Abuse: Lessons for practice in Slater, P., and Eastman, M. (1999) (Eds.), *Elder Abuse: Critical Issues in Policy and Practice*, London, Age Concern Books.

Penhale, B., and Kingston, P. (1995) Social Perspectives on Elder Abuse in Kingston, P., and Penhale, B. (1995) (Eds.), *Family Violence and the Caring Professions*. Basingstoke, Macmillan.

Penhale, B., and Parker, J. (1999) Older Men and Elder Abuse in *Seminar Proceedings: Men and Violence against Women*, Strasbourg, Council of Europe, EG/SEM/VIO (99) 21.

Phillipson, C. (1982) *Capitalism and the Construction of Old Age*. London, Macmillan.

Phillipson, C. (1992) Confronting Elder Abuse, *Generations Review*, 2, (3), 2-3.

Phillipson, C. (1993) Abuse of Older People: Sociological Perspectives in Decalmer, P., and Glendenning, F. (Eds.), (1993). *The Mistreatment of Elderly People*, London, Sage.

Pillemer, K. A., and Wolf, R. S. (Eds.). (1986). *Elder Abuse: conflict in the Family*, Dover, MA, Auburn House.

Pillemer, K. A., and Finkelhor, D. (1988) The prevalence of elder abuse: A random sample survey, *Gerontologist*, 28 (1): 51-57.

Pillemer, K. A., and Suitor, J. (1988) Elder Abuse in Van Hasselt, V., Morrison, R., Belack, A., and Hensen, M. (1988). (Eds.), *Handbook of Family Violence*, New York, Plenum Press.

Pritchard, J. (1992) *The Abuse of Elderly People: A Handbook for Professionals*, London, Jessica Kingsley.

Pritchard, J. (2000) *The Needs of Older Women: Services for victims of elder abuse and other abuse*, Bristol: The Policy Press.

Pritchard, J. (2001) *The Abuse of Older Men*, London, Jessica Kingsley.

Schaffer, J. (1999) Older and Isolated Women and Domestic Violence Project *Journal of Elder Abuse & Neglect*, 11, (1), 59-78.

Sengstock, M. (1991) Sex and gender implications in elder abuse, *Journal of Women & Aging*, 3, (2), 25-43.

Stearns, P. (1986) Old Age Family Conflict: The Perspective of the Past, In Pillemer, K. A., and Wolf, R.S. (Eds.), *Elder Abuse: Conflict in the Family*, Dover MA, Auburn House.

Steuer, J., and Austin, E. (1980) Family Abuse of the Elderly, *Journal of the American Geriatrics Society*, 28, (8), 372-376.

Stevenson, O., and Parsloe, P. (1993) *Community Care and Empowerment*, York: Joseph Rowntree Foundation.

Tatara, T. (1993) Finding the nature and scope of domestic elder abuse with state aggregate data, *Journal of Elder Abuse & Neglect*, 5, (4), 35-58.

Teaster, P., Roberto, K., Duke, J., and Kim, M. (2000) Sexual Abuse of Older Adults: Preliminary findings of cases in Virginia, *Journal of Elder Abuse & Neglect*, 12, (3/4), 1-16.

Townsend, P. (1981) The Structured Dependency of the Elderly: The Creation of Social Policy in the Twentieth Century. *Ageing and Society*, 1, (1), 5-28.

United States House of Representatives, Select Committee on Aging (1981) *Elder Abuse: The Hidden Problem*. Washington, DC: US Government Printing Office.

Vinton, L. (1992) Battered Women's Shelters and Older Women: The Florida Experience, *Journal of Family Violence*, 7, (1), 63-72

Walker, A. (1986) Pensions and the Production of Poverty in Old Age. In Phillipson, C., and Walker, A. (Eds.), *Ageing and Social Policy: A Critical Assessment*. Aldershot, Gower.

Whalen, M. (1996) *Counseling to End Violence Against Women: A Subversive Model*, Thousand Oaks, Sage.

Whittaker, T. (1995a) Violence, Gender and elder abuse: Towards a feminist analysis and practice, *Journal of Gender Studies*, 4, (1), 35-45.

Whittaker, T. (1995b) Gender and elder abuse in Arber, S., and Ginn, J. (1995) (Eds.), *Connecting gender and ageing: Sociological approaches to gender relations in later life*, Buckingham, Open University Press.

Wolf, R. (1993) Responding to elder abuse in the USA, *Action on Elder Abuse Working paper No. 1: A Report of the proceedings of the 1st International Symposium on elder abuse*. London, Action on Elder Abuse.

Wolf, R.S., and Pillemer, K.A. (1989) *Helping Elderly Victims: The reality of elder abuse*. New York, Columbia University Press.

Elder Abuse Risk Indicators
and Screening Questions:
Results from a Literature Search
and a Panel of Experts
from Developed and Developing Countries

Christen L. Erlingsson, RN, MScN
Sharon L. Carlson, RN, PhD, CNS
Britt-Inger Saveman, RNT, PhD, FEANS

Christen L. Erlingsson is Doctoral Candidate and University Lecturer, Department of Health and Behavioral Sciences, University of Kalmar, 391 82 Kalmar, Sweden (E-mail: christen.erlingsson@hik.se). Sharon L. Carlson is Professor, Nursing Department, Otterbein College, One Otterbein College, Westerville, OH 43081 USA (E-mail: scarlson@otterbein.edu). Britt-Inger Saveman is Associate Professor, Department of Health and Behavioral Sciences, University of Kalmar, 391 82 Kalmar, Sweden (E-mail: britt-inger.saveman@hik.se).

Address correspondence to: Christen L. Erlingsson at the above address.

The authors would like to thank the members in the Delphi panel for participating in the study and Kalmar University, the World Health Organization (WHO) and the International Network for the Prevention of Elder Abuse and Neglect (INPEA) for financial support.

[Haworth co-indexing entry note]: "Elder Abuse Risk Indicators and Screening Questions: Results from a Literature Search and a Panel of Experts from Developed and Developing Countries." Erlingsson, Christen L., Sharon L. Carlson, and Britt-Inger Saveman. Co-published simultaneously in *Journal of Elder Abuse & Neglect* (The Haworth Maltreatment & Trauma Press, an imprint of The Haworth Press, Inc.) Vol. 15, No. 3/4, 2003, pp. 185-203; and: *Elder Abuse: Selected Papers from the Prague World Congress on Family Violence* (ed: Elizabeth Podnieks, Jordan I. Kosberg, and Ariela Lowenstein) The Haworth Maltreatment & Trauma Press, an imprint of The Haworth Press, Inc., 2003, pp. 185-203. Single or multiple copies of this article are available for a fee from The Haworth Document Delivery Service [1-800-HAWORTH, 9:00 a.m. - 5:00 p.m. (EST). E-mail address: docdelivery@haworthpress.com].

SUMMARY. In order to examine and compare expert opinions from elder abuse literature on risk indicators and screening questions to perspectives of experts from both developed and developing countries, a literature search was combined with a modified Delphi process involving 17 panel members. Each method resulted in a consensus on 48 risk indicators. These shared only 35% content. Each method also resulted in a consensus on screening questions: Thirteen questions for the literature search and nine for the Delphi panel. There were divergences between Delphi panel participants' responses from developed and developing countries indicating that more research is needed in developing countries. *[Article copies available for a fee from The Haworth Document Delivery Service: 1-800-HAWORTH. E-mail address: <docdelivery@haworthpress.com> Website: <http://www.HaworthPress.com> © 2003 by The Haworth Press, Inc. All rights reserved.]*

KEYWORDS. Elder abuse, risk indicators, screening

BACKGROUND

Although ideally positioned to detect abuse of elders (American Medical Association, 1992; Aravanis et al., 1993), many health care practitioners throughout the world are ill equipped to identify elder abuse (O'Brien, 1996). The lack of a professional protocol for detection has been suggested to be a barrier to elder abuse identification (Krueger & Patterson, 1997). A call for detection instruments in health care settings has been expressed in international literature (Davies, 1997c; Fulmer & O'Malley, 1987; Kosberg & Garcia, 1995; Saveman & Sandvide, 2001). Particularly, there is a need for reliable, brief, and time efficient instruments for use in primary care in all countries, whether developed or developing (Davies, 1997c; Lachs, 1995; O'Brien, 1996; Rosenblatt, Cho, & Durance, 1996). However, there are no universally accepted standardized detection instruments available today (Rosenblatt, 1996). Prerequisite to development of a standardized protocol for worldwide use there is a need to structure and clarify cultural commonalities and consistencies as well as recognize cultural differences and divergences.

The World Health Organization (WHO) and the International Network for the Prevention of Elder Abuse and Neglect (INPEA) have stated the need for global detection instruments. The Global Response Against Elder Abuse Together (GREAT) is a joint project of the WHO and INPEA. One of the keystones in the GREAT project is the development of elder abuse detection instrument prototypes to be piloted in primary care contexts in developing countries.

Eighty percent of the one million people who live in the developing world turn 60 years of age each month. The proportion of older people is expected to more than double in developing countries by the year 2020. At the same time, developing countries are experiencing economic and social changes such as urbanization and changes in family. These changes, demographic, economic and social, together with existing inequality and poverty, create situations where elder abuse can proliferate (World Health Organization/International Network for the Prevention of Elder Abuse, 2002). There is no established definition or consensus on what entails a "developed" or "developing" country. In common practice, though, countries of Europe, Canada, the United States, Japan, Australia, and New Zealand are considered developed countries or regions (United Nations, 2003).

Primary care is a diverse concept and is organized in a variety of ways in both developed and developing countries around the globe. The breadth of integration among various primary health care occupations also varies intra- and internationally. The WHO/INPEA elder abuse detection instrument prototypes will be designed for use by clinicians in traditional clinical settings while remaining flexible enough to be adaptable for use by other professionals and in other settings outside the clinic (e.g., visiting nurses and social workers). The use of standardized detection documentation, a cornerstone of all healthcare activity, will help ensure adequate screening, facilitate development of a care plan, and simplify communication between disciplines in order to provide coordinated care for older people (Rosenblatt, 1996). Key ingredients in elder abuse detection documentation are risk indicators. Risk indicators have been described as predictive of the presence of abuse or an abusive situation (Hwalek & Sengstock, 1986). An awareness of risk indicators is considered to assist the practitioner to make connections to signs, symptoms, and behaviors of abuse (Nagpaul, 2001).

This paper describes the first step needed to develop specific instruments for detection of elder abuse. This first step involves a literature search combined with a modified Delphi process. These two methods will result in identification of consensuses and divergences. The aim of this paper is to examine and compare expert opinions from elder abuse literature on risk indicators and screening questions to perspectives of experts who are members of an international Delphi panel.

METHODOLOGY

Literature Search

In order to identify commonalities in existing elder abuse literature, a literature search focusing on risk indicators and screening questions concerning abuse of elders was performed. This search was initiated by disseminating a networking letter via e-mail to INPEA and WHO contacts. The letter was a request for known literature, new and unpublished studies, as well as for information on projects in progress. The letter was intended to snowball into each letter recipient's network, harvesting information not available through more traditional search forms. Time frame for the literature search through the networking letter occurred during a four-month period in the middle of 2002.

A literature search was also conducted which combined a database search and a search of the World Wide Web. The database search for scientific literature was based primarily on searches of Medline, CINAHL, ERIC, PyschINFO, EBSCO, and Elsevier. Search words and MESH terms were used according to each database thesaurus and included *elder abuse, elder mistreatment, protocol, assessment,* and *screening*. These terms were used independently, truncated, and in combinations with each other. Additional sources were located after hand searching the reference lists from identified literature. Searches of the World Wide Web were conducted using search engines such as Google, Alta Vista, and Yahoo. Search words used on the World Wide Web were the same as in the database search but were expanded to add the words *guidelines, domestic violence, adult abuse, body maps,* and Adult Protection Services as *APS*. The database and World Wide Web search was conducted during the same period as the networking letter.

It is important to emphasize that the literature search was not conducted in order to review and evaluate the evidence found, but the goal of the search was to be as comprehensive as possible during the identified search time frame in order to assess what information was currently available. No limitations were set on the age of the material. Quality of the pages from the World Wide Web was reviewed by examining stated references, author's affiliations, or the organization represented on the home page. Since screening instruments were defined as a set of questions directed to the patient, other materials, e.g., checklists and home environment protocols, were not considered relevant as screening instruments in this study. Manifest content analysis (Berg, 2001) was used to categorize the relevant data.

Modified Delphi Process

The Delphi method was chosen to augment the literature search in a continuing attempt to identify common and divergent perspectives among another group of elder abuse experts. The Delphi technique is a process that uses a panel of experts responding to several rounds of questionnaires. Between each round, the researchers analyze the returned material, summarize the results, and prepare individualized feedback for each panel member. This process allows an opportunity for panel members to modify their answers keeping replies of other respondents in mind. The anonymity inherent in the procedure is considered to encourage greater frankness than would be the norm in a face-to-face meeting. The goal is to achieve a group consensus (Polit & Beck, 2004).

However, in this study modifications were made in order to be more compact and expedient than in a traditional Delphi approach. Specifically, these modifications reflected problems in computer/e-mail systems and time as well as funding limitations for the study. The modified Delphi process discussed in this paper involved two rounds. In Round One a two-part questionnaire was disseminated concerning risk indicators and screening questions identified through the literature search. The summary of the individual and group responses from the first round was disseminated in Round Two and resulted in the consensus opinion of the Delphi panel. An additional questionnaire, relevant for the development of an assessment instrument prototype, which is the next step in the WHO/INPEA project, will be described elsewhere.

Participants and Settings

Panel members were identified through WHO and INPEA contacts. There were 17 panel members, considered elder abuse experts, who agreed to participate: eleven women and six men. The Delphi panel included participants with various academic degrees although doctoral degrees dominated. The panel members represented various fields: medicine (n = 4), nursing (n = 4), sociology (n = 3), social work (n = 3), psychology (n = 2), and health management (n = 1). Panel members represented twelve countries including Argentina, Austria, Brazil, Canada, Chile, India, Lebanon, Kenya, Mozambique, Sweden, United Kingdom, and the USA. Contact with panel members was conducted using e-mail, fax, and ordinary mail. All panel members' responses were treated confidentially.

Questionnaire, Data Collection, and Analysis

The modified Delphi process was conducted during the fall of 2002. An information letter was sent to panel members at the start of each of the rounds. Panel members were encouraged to respond to a two-part questionnaire using their own cultural framework for reference.

The risk indicators identified from the literature search were used as the basis for the first part of the questionnaire. Many indicators were similar and therefore combined, e.g., "cuts" was combined with "lacerations" and "broken bones" combined with "fractures." Other items, although referred to in the original source as a risk indicator proved to be signs of actual abuse and were deleted, e.g., "Caretaker threatens the elder with punishment." The remaining risk indicators were presented in the first part of the questionnaire. Panel members were asked to decide if each item (n = 263) should be included or discarded from the ongoing Delphi process. Items chosen for inclusion were to be rated as "high risk," "medium risk," or "low risk" indicators of elder abuse. Space was provided on the questionnaire for comments.

The second part of the questionnaire contained questions for screening for elder abuse. Many of the screening questions found through the literature search were also similar. Because there were differences in wording, which inferred significant subtleties in meaning, all identified screening questions (n = 67) were included in the second part of the questionnaire. Again, the panel members were asked to choose which questions they believed should be included that best captured nuances of elder abuse.

Data from Round One were analyzed both at the individual participant and group levels and disseminated in Round Two as an individualized feedback highlighting personal responses for comparison against responses of other panel members. In Round Two each panel member also had the opportunity to review their individual responses and to change their initial responses after this review. Those risk indicator items rated highest by the entire panel were included in a consensus list. Cluster analyses of the Round One data were performed using SPSS 11.0.

RESULTS

Results will be presented according to the sequence used in the methodological process. First a presentation of the commonalities seen in the literature search will be presented and then the consensus and divergent results from the Delphi Panel Rounds One and Two will be described. Finally, the commonalities and divergences between the literature search and the Delphi panel opinions will be presented.

Literature Search

The networking letter yielded one elder abuse protocol. In addition there were 182 sources located through both the database and World Wide Web searches. The literature search was focused to identify current opinions on *risk indicators* and *screening questions* held by experts as a group. There were 31 sources selected for review of content for *risk indicators* of elder abuse and 24 sources selected for review of content for *screening questions* (references marked with an asterisk in the reference list indicate studies included in the results of the literature search). The remaining material included content on assessment instruments (n = 50), to be described elsewhere, or was of a more general character providing additional background information. In the 31 sources selected for review of *risk indicator* content, 565 risk indicators were identified; most of these were located in checklists that were the basis for detection instruments. The *risk indicators* mentioned in five or more references (n = 48) were included in a literature search consensus list (see Table 1).

In the 24 sources with content on *screening questions* for elder abuse, 17 instruments were identified, five of which were domestic violence screening instruments applicable to cases of elder abuse. There were 67 discrete *screening questions* identified. Many of these questions combined different aspects of abuse in the same question. An example of this combination is the question, "Has anyone at home ever hurt you?" which could be considered a question on physical, sexual, and psychological abuse. There were 13 questions repeated in three or more sources representing a consensus of *screening questions* identified through the literature search (see Table 2). The results of the literature search showed that research on *risk indicators* and *screening questions* in the field of elder abuse almost exclusively has been conducted in developed countries.

The Delphi Panel

Results from Round One

Of 17 selected panel members, 12 responded to the risk indicator items (n = 263) and 10 responded to the *screening items* (n = 67). Dendrograms based on responses to *risk indicator items* confirmed a distinct trend for panel members (n = 5) from developed countries to answer in a like manner. Also answers from respondents from developing countries (n = 7) were clustered together. It is noteworthy that these two trends in responses concerning *risk indicators* only related to whether the respondent came from developed or developing countries. An example of this is that panel members (n = 5) from developed countries rated the item, "Caregiver ill prepared to give care" as "low risk" for elder abuse, while all seven panel members from developing countries rated that specific item as "high risk" for abuse of elders.

The divergent responses between panel members from developed and developing countries continued to be evident in results of the *screening items*. An example of this is that four of the five panel members from developed countries considered the *screening question* "Who cares for you at home?" as non-relevant, while all five panel members from developing countries considered it relevant and important. Again divergence between panel members from developed and developing countries could be seen.

Results from Round Two

The same 12 panel members responded to the *risk indicator items* in Round Two. Results regarding *risk indicator items* (n = 263) revealed

TABLE 1. Risk Indicators Consensus Between Literature Search and Delphi Panel, and Risk Indicators Unique to Literature Search and Delphi Panel.

	General indicators
Risk indicators common to both literature search consensus and Delphi panel consensus	History of family violence (violence normal response to stress) Drug or alcohol addiction in family Excessive dependence of elder or caregiver Reports of being left in an unsafe situation Poor past relationship/poor current relationship (issues of power, control, coercion, dominance, or manipulation)
Risk indicators unique to the literature search consensus	History of untreated psychiatric problems in elder or caregiver Noncompliance Therapeutic failure Prolonged interval between injury and medical treatment Inadequate food supply History of doctor hopping
Risk indicators unique to Delphi panel consensus	Evidence of unusual family stress/recent family crisis

	Indicators specific for the abused elder	Indicators specific for the abuser
Risk indicators common to both literature search consensus and Delphi panel consensus	Isolation of elder Physical impairment of older adult	Financially dependent on elder Gives vague, implausible, inconsistent, or no explanations for elder's injuries Substance abuse (alcohol and drugs) Hostility
Risk indicators unique to the literature search consensus	Exhibits fearful behavior Poor hygiene Depression Living with relatives Acute and chronic health problems Confusion Withdrawal	Has mental illness Poor finances A blamer Depression Loss of job Ill prepared to give care Frustrated Poor health Poor knowledge of patient's medical problems
Risk indicators unique to Delphi panel consensus	Victim of past abuse Substance abuse (alcohol or drugs) Fearfulness towards caregiver	Lack of resources, e.g., time, money, energy History of violence, abuse, neglect, or exploitation Current violence towards family members or pets Intolerance of the older person's behavior Perception of stress as a load too heavy to bear/overwhelmed Is forced by circumstances to care for the patient who is unwanted Aggressive Dependent on the abused Denies access to client

	Indicators of physical abuse	Indicators of sexual abuse	Indicators of financial abuse
Risk indicators common to both literature search consensus and Delphi panel consensus	Fractures in various stages of healing Friction from ropes or chains Dehydration Injuries in shape of object that inflicted them Unexplained burns Cigar/cigarette burns	(none)	(none)
Risk indicators unique to the literature search consensus	Unexplained bruises Malnourishment Bruises in various stages of healing Contractures Absence of hair Decubitis Broken nose or teeth	Bleeding Bruising on inner thigh	(none)

TABLE 1 (continued)

	Indicators of physical abuse	Indicators of sexual abuse	Indicators of financial abuse
Risk indicators unique to Delphi panel consensus	Unexplained injuries Injuries or traumas inconsistent with reported causes Multiple injuries Signs of hair pulling (hemorrhaging below scalp) Slap marks Suspicious falls or injuries Previous similar injuries Fractures in unusual locations Marks left by gag Injuries in unusual locations Black eyes Bruises not consistent with a fall	Trauma to: Genitals Breasts Rectum Mouth	Evidence that personal belongings of elder are being taken without elder's consent Unexplained loss of social security/ pension checks

that the five panel members from the developed countries did not consider any indicators as "high risk"; 6% of the items were rated as "medium risk"; and 65% of the items as "low risk" for elder abuse. The panel members from developed countries considered 29% of the items as non-relevant. In contrast, all seven panel members from the developing countries rated 2% of the items as "high risk," 49% of the items as "medium risk" and 48% of them as "low risk" for elder abuse. Further, these panel members considered all items relevant and important.

Concerning *screening questions*, the five panel members from developed countries included only 24 of the identified *screening questions*, while the five panel members from the developing countries chose to include 54 *screening questions*. There was consensus between panel members from both developed and developing countries on nine questions, with only one question in common (see Table 2).

Commonalities and Divergences Between the Literature Search Results and the Modified Delphi Panel Results

Both risk indicator consensuses and screening question consensuses arise from experts' opinions found in the literature search and the Delphi panel responses. The risk indicator consensus lists from the literature search and the modified Delphi process (see Table 1) had 35% of risk indicators in common. Consensus elements shared by both the liter-

TABLE 2. Consensus Lists of Screening Questions from the Literature Search and the Delphi Panel

Literature search	Delphi panel
1. Are you afraid of anyone at home?	1. Who makes decisions about your life, such as how or where you will live?
2. Are you alone a lot?	
3. Has anyone ever touched you without your consent?	2. Has anyone ever hit, slapped, restrained, or hurt you physically?
4. Has anyone ever made you do things you didn't want to do?	3. Do you need help taking care of yourself?
5. Has anyone at home ever hurt you?	4. Has anyone ever withheld food or medications from you?
6. Has anyone ever scolded or threatened you?	5. Does your caregiver depend on you for shelter or money?
7. Have you signed any documents that you didn't understand?	6. Has anyone touched you sexually without your permission?
8. Do you take your own medications?	7. Does anyone at home make you uncomfortable or afraid?
9. Are you punished in any way?	
10. Has anyone ever withheld food or medications from you?	8. Has anyone forced you to do something that you did not understand, such as sign documents?
11. Do you support anyone?	
12. Has anyone taken anything that was yours without asking?	9. Has anyone ever failed to help you take care of yourself when you needed help?
13. Has anyone ever failed to help you take care of yourself when you needed help?	

ature search and the modified Delphi process included: (1) a history of violence and addiction, (2) an isolated and physically impaired abused elder, (3) a hostile abuser, and (4) fractures, dehydration, burns, etc., indicating physical abuse. The differences between results from the literature search and from the Delphi panel could be seen for example in risk indicators for sexual and financial abuse (see Table 1). Screening questions differed in number between consensus in the literature search results and consensus of the Delphi panel responses. Although variance is evident in wordings of questions, the essential meaning of the screening questions in these two consensuses may be considered similar. The screening questions were dissimilar in that the questions in the literature search consensus were general and indirect with, e.g., sexual abuse implicit in the wordings. In contrast the questions selected through the modified Delphi process were direct questions including an explicit question on sexual abuse (see Table 2).

DISCUSSION

The literature search on detection of elder abuse combined a database search, World Wide Web search and information found through a networking letter. All of the data resulting from the search originated in developed countries. The literature search resulted in the identification of 565 risk indicators and 67 discrete screening questions. In addition, a modified Delphi process was conducted where panel members from 12 countries indicated preferences for risk indicator items and screening questions for detecting elder abuse. Evident in the results from panel member selections was a divergence between choices made by members from developed and developing countries.

From the risk indicators unique to the literature search consensus and to the Delphi panel consensus (see Table 1); two different pictures about the abused elder and the abuser emerged. A picture drawn from the literature search consensus shows an abused elder who exhibits fearful and depressive behaviors. The abused elder also has acute or chronic health problems, is confused and withdrawn. This person lives with relatives and has poor hygiene. The abuser in this picture has poor health, mental illness, and depression. The abuser is unemployed, and a blamer, is ill prepared to give care and has inadequate knowledge of the elder's medical problems. Both the abused and the abuser seem to be in a "no win situation." The abused elder needs support and help but the abuser has limited resources to provide the needed assistance. It is also out of this environment that abuse arises, a situation where both the abused and the abuser need help.

A picture drawn from the consensus risk indicators from the modified Delphi process show the abused elder as a substance abuser and a victim of past abuse. This person is fearful of the caregiver. The abuser in this picture has a history of violence and continues this pattern. This person lacks energy, time, and money but is forced by circumstances to care for the elder. The abuser also is overwhelmed by stress, has an intolerance of the elder's behavior, and yet denies any access by others to the elder. Abuse in this case may arise from the personality of the abuser and the structure of a society that expects the family to care for its elders. This idea is supported by Saveman, Hallberg, and Norberg (1996), who found through interviews with professional caregivers, that family caregivers were not always suited to give care, yet felt an obligation from society to care for elderly relatives.

The results from the Delphi panel risk indicator consensus may reflect the culture, traditions, and societal expectations found in any country where family is expected to provide for their elders. The results from the literature search, which came from developed countries, together with the results from the Delphi panel, which included experts from developing countries, suggest that more studies need to be done in order to better understand cultural factors that are associated with elder abuse in developing countries in contrast to developed countries.

The literature search consensus revealed a general preference for the use of risk indicators in checklists. Although there could be several advantages to using checklists, e.g., a time saving way for documentation not necessarily involving a patient interview, it is questionable whether checklists of risk indicators, e.g., "Bruises," "Depression," "Weight loss," can be efficiently used without previous education and training in elder abuse detection. A health professional's lack of education in the field of elder abuse is considered a barrier to detection (Clarke & Pierson, 1999; Lachs, 1995; Noone & Decalmer; 1997, O'Brien, 1996; Saveman & Sandvide, 2001). Education is also often required to be able to judge if observed symptoms are signs of aging or if abuse should be suspected (Hirsch, Stratton, Loewry, 1999; O'Brien, 1996). Until further research is conducted on risk indicators in developing countries, research results indicate the need for a training manual to accompany the detection instruments disseminated in the developing world.

The literature search consensus list included screening questions using a variety of question formats, often involving multiple types of abuse within one and the same question. In comparison, the Delphi panel consensus list included only one question that could be interpreted as involving multiple types of abuse. This one question was also included in the literature search consensus list. The remaining questions chosen by the Delphi panel were direct questions (see Table 2). There are varying opinions about the kind of questions that are best to use in screening for elder abuse. Some authors recommend the initial use of general, open-ended questions, leading to more specific questions (e.g., Clarke & Pierson, 1999; Lachs & Pillemer, 1995; O'Brien, 1996; Quinn & Tomita, 1997). In contrast, more direct questions are recommended by other authors (e.g., American Medical Association, 1992; Aravanis et al., 1993; Butler, 1999; Haviland & O'Brien, 1989), although open- ended questions are also suggested (e.g., Hirsch & Loewy, 2001; Ramsey-Klawsnik, 1996). Further research is needed to determine which types of screening questions are most appropriate to use in developing countries. The opinions voiced by Delphi panel members in this study indicate that direct questions should be utilized.

The literature search consensus on risk indicators was based on those indicators shown to be most commonly occurring in the literature. As Ansello (1996) points out, "Although sheer repetition [*of risk indicators*] does not confer credibility, it does carry weight in defining the debate . . . " (p. 15). There are seven risk indicators considered to be validated through scientific studies including indicators specific for the abused (shared living, social isolation, and dementia) and indicators specific for the abuser (mental illness, hostility, alcohol abuse, and dependency of the abuser on the abused) (National Research Council, 2003). These seven validated risk indicators, however, only begin to encompass the diverse and complex field of detecting elder abuse. Whether these same seven are valid in both developed and developing countries remains to be seen. Identifying a set of risk indicators suggest an opportunity for early intervention (Shugarman, Fries, Wolf, & Morris, 2003). There is today no established consensus on a list of risk indicators (Shugarman, Fries, Wolf, & Morris, 2003) that otherwise could be utilized in the development of global instruments for detection of elder abuse.

It can be argued that, despite participation by panel members from developing countries, the results still only reflected the risk indicator items and screening questions that in turn originated in material from developed countries. Providing space on the questionnaire for comments hopefully mitigated this fact. However, panel members suggested no new questions and few alternative risk indicators were suggested. These risk indicators were so similar to items that had already been discarded by the panel that they were not included in the continuing modified Delphi process.

The method used with networking letter, literature search and a modified Delphi process has limitations. The researchers could not control the networking letter's efficiency. It cannot be known if there actually are no research or grass roots programs for detection of elder abuse in developing countries or if the absence of feedback was more due to disinterest or lack of knowledge on the part of letter recipients. Another limitation was the small number of participants on the Delphi panel which limits the generalizability of the results (Polit & Beck, 2004). It is also unknown to the researchers why some panel members answered only parts of the questionnaire. The time limitations for the study might have contributed to the missing data. Yet keeping in mind that the modified Delphi process aimed to incorporate opinions from developing countries, the present results, especially in light of the divergence between panel members from developed and developing countries could be considered to have fulfilled the goal.

CONCLUSION

The differences between the two sets of consensuses (literature search and modified Delphi process) as well as the divergent results seen between the Delphi panel members from developed and developing countries are yet another wake-up call that more elder abuse research is needed in developing countries.

REFERENCES

References marked with an asterisk indicate studies included in the results of the literature search.

Ansello, E. F. (1996). Causes and theories. In L. A. Baumhover, & S. C. Beall (Eds.), *Abuse, Neglect, and Exploitation of Older Persons: Strategies for Assessment and Intervention* (pp. 9-29). Baltimore: Health Professions Press.

*American Medical Association. (1992). *Diagnostic and treatment guidelines on elder abuse and neglect.* Chicago: Author.

*Aravanis, S. C., Adelman, R. D., Breckman, R., Fulmer, T. T., Holder, E., Lachs, M., et al. (1993). Diagnostic and treatment guidelines on elder abuse and neglect. *Archives of Family Medicine, 2*(4), 371-388.

*Bass, D., Anetzberger, G., Ejaz, F., & Nagpaul, K. (2001). Screening tools and referral protocol for stopping abuse against older Ohioans: A guide for service providers. *Journal of Elder Abuse & Neglect, 13*(2), 23-38.

Berg, B. L. (2001). *Qualitative Research Methods for the Social Sciences* (4th ed.). Boston: Allyn & Bacon.

*Bloom, J. S., Ansell, P., & Bloom, M. N. (1989). Detecting elder abuse: A guide for physicians. *Geriatrics, 44*(6), 40-44.

*Breckman, R. S., & Adelman, R. D. (1988). *Strategies for Helping Victims of Elder Mistreatment.* Newbury Park, CA: Sage Publications.

*Butler, R. N. (1999). Warning signs of elder abuse. *Geriatrics, 54*(3), 3-4.

*Clarke, M. E., & Pierson, W. (1999). Management of elder abuse in the emergency department. *Emergency Medicine Clinics of North America, 17*(3), 631-644.

*Choi, N. G., & Mayer, J. (2000). Elder abuse, neglect, and exploitation: Risk factors and prevention strategies. *Journal of Gerontological Social Work, 33*(2), 5-25.

*Davies, M. (1997a). Appendix D: Elder abuse assessment protocol for nurses. In P. Decalmer, & F. Glendenning (Eds.), *The Mistreatment of Elderly People* (2nd ed.) (pp. 233-235). London: Sage Publications.

*Davies, M. (1997b). Appendix E: Carer abuse assessment protocol for nurses. In P. Decalmer, & F. Glendenning (Eds.), *The Mistreatment of Elderly People* (2nd ed.). (pp. 236-238). London: Sage Publications.

Davies, M. (1997c). Key issues for nursing: The need to challenge practice. In P. Decalmer, & F. Glendenning (Eds.), *The Mistreatment of Elderly People* (2nd ed.) (pp. 175-185). London: Sage Publications.

*Decalmer, P. (1997). Clinical presentation and management. In P. Decalmer, & F. Glendenning (Eds.), *The Mistreatment of Elderly People* (2nd ed.) (pp. 42-73). London: Sage Publications.

*DiLoreto, S. (2001). Domestic violence: Detection and treatment. *Patient Care, 35*(7), 68-88.

*Freutel, K. (n.d.). *R.I.S.C.: A program to improve the detection and management of elder abuse by family physicians.* London, Ontario: Author.

Fulmer, T. T., & O'Malley, T. A. (1987). *Inadequate Care of the Elderly: A Health Care Perspective on Abuse and Neglect*: New York: Springer Publications.

*Fulmer, T., Paveza, G., Abraham, I., & Fairchild, S. (2000). Elder neglect assessment in the emergency department. *Journal of Emergency Nursing, 26*(5), 436-443.

*Fulmer, T., & Wetle, T. (1986). Elder abuse screening and intervention. *Nurse Practitioner, 11*(5), 33-38.

*Gray-Vickrey, P. (2001). Protecting the older adult. *Nursing Management, 32*(10), 36-40.

*Hamilton, G. P. (1989). Prevent elder abuse-using a family systems approach. *Journal of Gerontological Nursing, 15*(3), 21-26.

*Haviland, S., & O'Brien, J. (1989). Physical abuse and neglect of the elderly: Assessment and intervention. *Orthopaedic Nursing, 8*(4), 11-19.

*Healthcare Providers Service Organization (HPSO). (n.d.). *When you suspect elder abuse.* Retrieved July 25, 2002 from http://www.hpso.com/newsletters/7-99flash.html

*Hirsch, C. H., & Loewy, R. (2001). The management of elder mistreatment: The physician's role. *Wiener Klinische Wochenschrift, 113* (10), 384-392.

*Hirsch, C. H., Stratton, S., & Loewy, R. (1999). The primary care of elder mistreatment. *Western Journal of Medicine, 170*(6), 353-358.

*Hwalek, M., Goodrich, C., & Quinn, M. J. (1996). The role of risk factors in health care and adult protective services. In L. A. Baumhover, & S. C. Beall (Eds.), *Abuse, Neglect, and Exploitation of Older Persons: Strategies for Assessment and Intervention* (pp. 123-142). Baltimore: Health Professions Press.

*Hwalek, M., & Sengstock, M. (1986). Assessing the probability of abuse of the elderly: Toward development of a clinical screening instrument. *Journal of Applied Gerontology, 5*(2), 153-173.

*Johnson, T. F. (1991). *Elder Mistreatment: Deciding Who is at Risk.* New York: Greenwood Press.

*Jones, J., Dougherty, J., Schelble, D., & Cunningham, W. (1988). Emergency department protocol for the diagnosis and evaluation of geriatric abuse. *Annals of Emergency Medicine, 17*(10), 1006-1015.

*Kosberg, J. I. (1988). Preventing elder abuse: Identification of high risk factors prior to placement decisions. *Gerontologist, 28*(1), 43-50.

*Kosberg, J. I., & Garcia, J. L. (1995). Introduction to the book. In J. I. Kosberg, & J. L. Garcia (Eds.), *Elder Abuse: International and Cross-cultural Perspectives* (pp. 1-12). New York: The Haworth Press, Inc.

*Kosberg, J. I., & Nahmiash, D. (1996). Characteristics of victims and perpetrators and milieus of abuse and neglect. In L. A. Baumhover, & S. C. Beall (Eds.), *Abuse, Ne-*

glect, and Exploitation of Older Persons: Strategies for Assessment and Intervention (pp. 31-50). Baltimore: Health Professions Press.

*Krouse, L. H. (June 5, 2001). Elder Abuse. *eMedicine Journal*, 2(6). Retrieved August 1, 2002 from http://www.emedicine.com/emerg/topic160.htm

Krueger, P., & Patterson, C. (1997). Detecting and managing elder abuse: Challenges in primary care. The Research Subcommittee of the Elder Abuse and Self-Neglect Task Force of Hamilton-Wentworth. *Canadian Medical Association Journal, 157* (8), 1095-1100.

Lachs, M. S. (1995). Preaching to the unconverted: Educating physicians about elder abuse. *Journal of Elder Abuse & Neglect*, 7(4), 1-12.

*Lachs, M. S., & Pillemer, K. (1995). Abuse and neglect of elderly persons. *New England Journal of Medicine*, 332(7), 437-443.

*Lachs, M. S., Williams, C., O'Brien, S., Hurst, L., & Horwitz, R. (1997). Risk factors for reported elder abuse and neglect: A nine-year observational cohort study. *Gerontologist*, 37(4), 469-474.

*Lynch, S. H. (1997). Elder abuse: What to look for, how to intervene. *American Journal of Nursing*, 97(1), 26-32.

*Marshall, C. E., Benton, D., & Brazier, J. M. (2000). Elder abuse. Using clinical tools to identify clues of mistreatment. *Geriatrics*, 55(2), 42-44.

*McAllister, M. (2000). Domestic violence: A life-span approach to assessment and intervention. *Lippincott's Primary Care Practice*, 4(2), 174-192.

*Mendonca, J. D., Velamoor, V. R., & Sauve, D. (1996). Key features of maltreatment of the infirm elderly in home settings. *Canadian Journal of Psychiatry–Revue Canadienne de Psychiatrie*, 41(2), 107-113.

*Mount Sinai/Victim Service Agency Elder Abuse Project. (1988). *Elder mistreatment guidelines for health professionals: Detection, assessment, and intervention.* New York: Author.

*Murphy, N. (1994). *Resource and training kit for service providers: Abuse and neglect of older adults.* Health Programs and Services Branch Health Canada. Retrieved July 25, 2002 from http://www.hc-sc.gc.ca/hppb/familyviolence/html/1oldtrain.htm

Nagpaul, K. (2001). Application of elder abuse screening tools and referral protocol: Techniques and clinical considerations. *Journal of Elder Abuse & Neglect*, 13(2), 59-78.

National Research Council. (2003). *Elder Mistreatment: Abuse, Neglect, and Exploitation in an Aging America. Panel to Review Risk and Prevalence of Elder Abuse and Neglect.* Washington, DC: The National Academies Press.

*Neufeld, B. (1996). SAFE questions: Overcoming barriers to the detection of domestic violence. *American Family Physician*, 53(8), 2575-2580.

Noone, J. F., & Decalmer, P. (1997). The general practitioner and elder abuse. In P. Decalmer, & F. Glendenning (Eds.), *The Mistreatment of Elderly People* (2nd ed.) (pp. 186-198). London: Sage.

*O'Brien, J. (1996). Screening: A primary care clinician's perspective. In L. A. Baumhover, & S. C. Beall (Eds.), *Abuse, Neglect, and Exploitation of Older Persons: Strategies for Assessment and Intervention* (pp. 51-64). Baltimore: Health Professions Press.

*Patterson, C. (March, 27, 1998). *Secondary prevention of elder abuse*. Canadian Task Force on Preventive Health Care. Retrieved May 21, 2002 from http://www.ctfphc. org/Full_Text/Ch77full.htm

Polit, D., & Beck, C. (2004). *Nursing Research: Principles and Methods* (7th ed.). Philadelphia: Lippincott.

*Pritchard, J. (1995). *The Abuse of Older People: A Training Manual for Detection and Prevention* (2nd ed.). London: Jessica Kingsley Publishers.

*Quinn, M. J., & Tomita, S. K. (1997). *Elder Abuse and Neglect: Causes, Diagnosis, and Intervention Strategies* (2nd ed.). New York: Springer Publishing.

*Ramsey-Klawsnik, H. (1996). Assessing physical and sexual abuse in health care settings. In L. A. Baumhover, & S. C. Beall (Eds.), *Abuse, Neglect, and Exploitation of Older Persons: Strategies for Assessment and Intervention* (pp. 67-88). Baltimore: Health Professions Press.

*Ramsey-Klawsnik, H. (2000). Elder abuse offenders: A typology. *Generations, 24*(2), 17-22.

*Reay, A. M., & Browne, K. D. (2001). Risk factor characteristics in carers who physically abuse or neglect their elderly dependents. *Aging & Mental Health, 5*(1), 56-62.

*Reis, M., & Nahmiash, D. (1998). Validation of the indicators of abuse (IOA) screen. *Gerontologist, 38*(4), 471-480.

*Rosenblatt, D. (1996). Documentation. In L. A. Baumhover, & S. C. Beall (Eds.), *Abuse, Neglect, and Exploitation of Older Persons: Strategies for Assessment and Intervention* (pp. 145-162). Baltimore: Health Professions Press.

Rosenblatt, D. E., Cho, K. H., & Durance, P. W. (1996). Reporting mistreatment of older adults: The role of physicians. *Journal of the American Geriatrics Society, 44*(1), 65-70.

*San Francisco Medical Society. (n.d.). *Domestic Violence: A Practical Approach for Clinicians*. Retrieved August 5, 2002 from http://www.sfms.org/broschure.htm

Saveman, B. I., Hallberg, I. R., & Norberg, A. (1996). Narratives by district nurses about elder abuse within families. *Clinical Nursing Research–An International Journal, 5*(2), 220-236.

Saveman, B. I., & Sandvide, A. (2001). Swedish general practitioners' awareness of elderly patients at risk of or actually suffering from elder abuse. *Scandinavian Journal of Caring Sciences, 15*(3), 244-249.

*Sengstock, M., & Steiner, S. (1996). Assessing non-physical abuse. In L. A. Baumhover, & S. C. Beall (Eds.), *Abuse, Neglect, and Exploitation of Older Persons: Strategies for Assessment and Intervention* (pp. 105-122). Baltimore: Health Professions Press.

*Sherin, K., Sinacore, J., Li, X. Q., Zitter, R., & Shakil, A. (1998). HITS: A short domestic violence screening tool for use in a family practice setting. *Family Medicine, 30*(7), 508-512.

Shugarman, L. R., Fries, B. E., Wolf, R. S., & Morris, J. N. (2003). Identifying older people at risk of abuse during routine screening practices. *Journal of the American Geriatrics Society, 51*, 24-31.

United Nations. (2003). *Definition of developed, developing countries*. Retrieved September 21, 2003 from http://unstats.un.org/unsd/mi/mi_dict_xrxx.asp?def_code=491

*Weiss, S., Garza, A., Casaletto, J., Stratton, M., Ernst, A., Blanton, D. et al. (2000). The out-of-hospital use of a domestic violence screen for assessing patient risk. *Prehospital Emergency Care, 4*(1), 24-27.

*Willson, P. (1998). Domestic violence: Are nurses hiding the facts? *Internet Journal of Advanced Nursing Practice, 2*(1). Retrieved June 7, 2002 from http://www.ispub. com/ostia/index.php?xmlFilePath=journals/ijanp/vol2n1/violence.xml

*Wolfe, S. (1998). Look for signs of abuse. *RN, 61*(8), 48-51.

World Health Organization/International Network for the Prevention of Elder Abuse. (2002). *Missing Voices: Views of Older Persons on Elder Abuse.* Geneva: World Health Organization.

*Woolard, R., & Bernstein, E. (n.d.). *Elder Abuse.* Society for Academic Emergency Medicine (S.A.E.M.). Retrieved July 25, 2002 from http://www.saem.org/inform/ eldabuse.htm

Index

BOOK ORDER FORM!

Order a copy of this book with this form or online at:
http://www.haworthpress.com/store/product.asp?sku=5516

Elder Abuse

Selected Papers from the Prague World Congress on Family Violence

_____ in softbound at $29.95 ISBN: 0-7890-2824-7.
_____ in hardbound at $49.95 ISBN: 0-7890-2823-9.

COST OF BOOKS _____

POSTAGE & HANDLING _____
US: $4.00 for first book & $1.50
for each additional book
Outside US: $5.00 for first book
& $2.00 for each additional book.

SUBTOTAL _____
In Canada: add 7% GST. _____

STATE TAX _____
CA, IL, IN, MN, NJ, NY, OH & SD residents
please add appropriate local sales tax.

FINAL TOTAL _____
If paying in Canadian funds, convert
using the current exchange rate,
UNESCO coupons welcome.

❑ BILL ME LATER:
Bill-me option is good on US/Canada/
Mexico orders only; not good to jobbers,
wholesalers, or subscription agencies.

❑ Signature _____

❑ Payment Enclosed: $ _____

❑ PLEASE CHARGE TO MY CREDIT CARD:
❑ Visa ❑ MasterCard ❑ AmEx ❑ Discover
❑ Diner's Club ❑ Eurocard ❑ JCB

Account # _____

Exp Date _____

Signature _____
(Prices in US dollars and subject to change without notice.)

PLEASE PRINT ALL INFORMATION OR ATTACH YOUR BUSINESS CARD

Name

Address

City   State/Province   Zip/Postal Code

Country

Tel   Fax

E-Mail

May we use your e-mail address for confirmations and other types of information? ❑ Yes ❑ No We appreciate receiving
your e-mail address. Haworth would like to e-mail special discount offers to you, as a preferred customer.
We will never share, rent, or exchange your e-mail address. We regard such actions as an invasion of your privacy.

Order from your **local bookstore** or directly from
The Haworth Press, Inc. 10 Alice Street, Binghamton, New York 13904-1580 • USA
Call our toll-free number (1-800-429-6784) / Outside US/Canada: (607) 722-5857
Fax: 1-800-895-0582 / Outside US/Canada: (607) 771-0012
E-mail your order to us: orders@haworthpress.com

For orders outside US and Canada, you may wish to order through your local
sales representative, distributor, or bookseller.
For information, see http://haworthpress.com/distributors

(Discounts are available for individual orders in US and Canada only, not booksellers/distributors.)

Please photocopy this form for your personal use.
www.HaworthPress.com   BOF05